MOVE • FEEL • THINK

YOGA
FOR BRAIN INJURY, PTSD AND OTHER FORMS OF TRAUMA

JANNA LEYDE

mft

The author and publisher cannot be held responsible for any injury, mishap, or damages incurred during the practice of exercises in this book. The author recommends consultation with a healthcare professional before beginning this or any other exercise program.

mft

Published by Move Feel Think
Printed in the United States of America

ISBN-13: 978-0990561248
ISBN-10: 0990561240
BISAC: Health/Fitness Yoga
Released: 11/01/2014

Illustrations by Nicole Ryan
Book Design by Emily Balawejder

Move Feel Think books may be ordered through booksellers, online at movefeelthink.com, or by contacting: Move Feel Think at movefeelthink@gmail.com.

This book would not be without my parents.

To my father, for his patience and practice.
To my mother, for her inspiration and ideas.

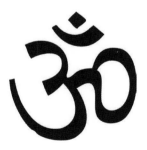

CONTENTS

FOREWARD

"AND NOW THE TEACHING ON YOGA BEGINS.

Yoga is the settling of the mind into silence.
When the mind has settled, we are established in our essential nature,
which is unbounded consciousness."
—Patanjali

These words introduce the original guide to yoga practice, *The Yoga Sutras of Patanjali*. While the exact origin of these collected aphorisms is often debated, their intent is not. The sutras describe the purpose and practice of yoga and its place in the journey toward *Samadhi*, or enlightenment. Western culture has focused on yoga as a purely physical pursuit; however, *The Yoga Sutras* clearly emphasizes the mental work that is required if one is to know the Self. Therefore, a yoga practice is an inquiry into the true nature of one's being, a personal journey inward on the path to self-awareness, and an affirmation and acceptance of what it is that frees the individual from the suffering imposed by the physical world. The yoga sutras teach us that yoga is much more than a set of physical poses that must be perfected. It is the mind that is the central focus of yoga, which makes yoga accessible to all, regardless of age, gender, race, religion, or physical state.

Today, science is beginning to embrace the mind-body connection and its central role in the mental and physical health of an individual, which is the exact message that *The Yoga Sutras of Patanjali* brought to mankind thousands of years ago. For individuals who live with traumatic brain injury, even the simplest of actions — brushing one's teeth, writing a check, finding the way home, saying hello, remembering a child's birthday or the names of loved ones —can be difficult if not impossible. Self-doubt, depression, and anxiety are often the byproducts of brain injury, and for patients with altered self-awareness and cognitive dysfunction, this often leads to despair, hopelessness, and a sense that control over one's life has been lost.

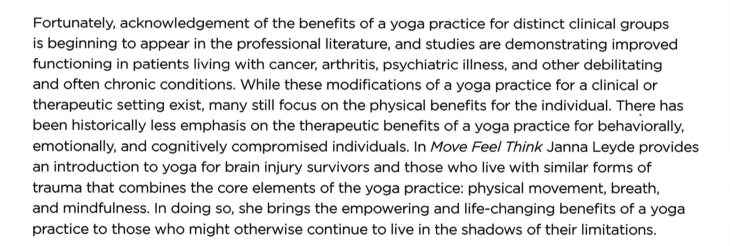

Fortunately, acknowledgement of the benefits of a yoga practice for distinct clinical groups is beginning to appear in the professional literature, and studies are demonstrating improved functioning in patients living with cancer, arthritis, psychiatric illness, and other debilitating and often chronic conditions. While these modifications of a yoga practice for a clinical or therapeutic setting exist, many still focus on the physical benefits for the individual. There has been historically less emphasis on the therapeutic benefits of a yoga practice for behaviorally, emotionally, and cognitively compromised individuals. In *Move Feel Think* Janna Leyde provides an introduction to yoga for brain injury survivors and those who live with similar forms of trauma that combines the core elements of the yoga practice: physical movement, breath, and mindfulness. In doing so, she brings the empowering and life-changing benefits of a yoga practice to those who might otherwise continue to live in the shadows of their limitations.

Janna's work is an inspiration to those who live with brain injury and trauma, the families who support and encourage them, and to anyone who is seeking a deeper understanding of the power of the mind-body connection.

Namaste,
Maryellen Romero, Ph.D.,
RYT
Clinical Neuropsychologist in the Department of Psychiatry and Behavioral Sciences
Tulane University School of Medicine, New Orleans, Louisiana

ONCE UPON A TIME I DIDN'T HAVE A REGULAR YOGA PRACTICE. Then a door opened and I walked into a hot, steamy studio nearly every single day during my two years of graduate school.

I thought yoga was physical. And it was. There were abs and arms to tone, weight to keep off, and toes to touch, but there was more. The bending, moving, and focusing was unearthing years of emotion. My practice was healing. I found myself craving yoga in place of food or drink, instead of closure and explanation. My practice was emotional medicine. Was I that sick? No, not really. I was lost and a little sad, hating a job I was supposed to love, and frustrated by life events gone wrong.

My father has a traumatic brain injury. His personality took the biggest blow in a car accident back in 1996, and we — my mom, me, our family, our friends — have struggled with his severe cognitive, emotional, and behavioral deficits ever since that day. Most things in his life require a prompt, a list, a plea. We are constantly reminding him to be more patient, more compassionate, more aware, less compulsive, less demanding, less angry. We're forever wading through the muck of challenges that come with his not being able to drive, work, or balance a bank account. It's an oscillation between failure and semi-success when it comes to recovering pieces of the "old John."

Yoga helped me understand, accept, and move past the fears and feelings that revolved around the inexplicable incident. By 2011, I had a year of certified yoga teaching under my belt (lesson: love something enough, make that something your career), and I had an inkling that yoga would help my father in ways that his cognitive and behavioral routines and treatments didn't. It was time to ask the right parties — my mother, his doctors.

My father and I began to practice together, and for the first time in 16 years we saw change — a renewed sense of purpose, a little more impulse control, self-discipline, and compassion toward others. Today my father's yoga practice continues to help him accept his mental and physical challenges and to embrace a more positive outlook. Yoga has helped him get back to the midline, to that place of balance, to that steady fulcrum we all crave.

I believe that yoga has a place in the brain injury treatment community. I believe that a routine yoga practice, like the one in this book, will enhance the lives of those who have lived through similar experiences, and I would like nothing more than to open that door to those who live with brain injury, post-traumatic stress disorder, and other forms of trauma.

Janna Leyde
the daughter.
the teacher.

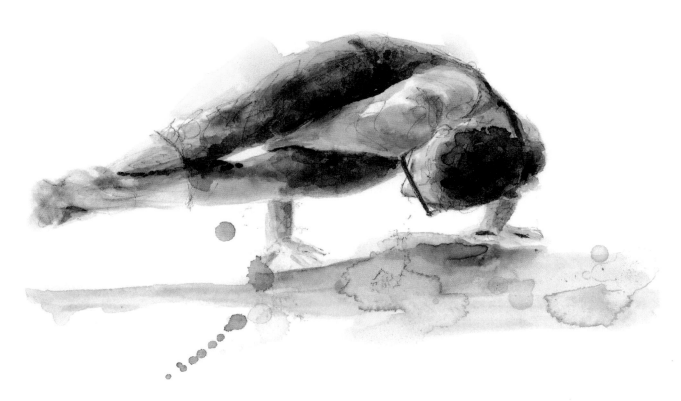

HOW CAN YOGA HELP A TRAUMA SURVIVOR?

WHAT IS YOGA?

Yoga means union. As translated from Sanskrit, yoga means **to yoke.** It is a practice that incorporates physical poses, breath work, and meditation to strengthen **the union between mind and body.**

Yoga is a holistic practice that can complement any lifestyle or current treatment plan. It focuses on the mind-body connection, allowing both aspects to benefit from one treatment modality. Yoga can be practiced independently or within a group session and is beneficial for both children and adults. **A routine yoga practice — set up for the specific individual, taking into consideration their capabilities — can make a notable, positive difference in his or her quality of life.**

HOW CAN YOGA HELP PEOPLE WHO LIVE WITH BRAIN INJURY OR PTSD?

The current yoga practices available to persons who live with brain injury, PTSD, and similar forms of trauma focus primarily on the physical body. These disciplines, such as Chair Yoga or Adaptive Yoga, are extremely healing for those who have lost mobility due to trauma and have helped individuals regain range of motion and decrease physical discomforts.

What else happens as a result of trauma? Not only is the physical body affected, but the mind-body connection is weakened or disconnected. Individuals who have sustained a trauma often experience a sense of displacement, loss of awareness, and lack of purpose, along with various emotional and intellectual challenges.

How can yoga help? Yoga is the movement of the physical body, yet even the most basic yoga poses engage the subtle body — or the energetic body. The subtle body is where one starts to build concepts, such as awareness, creativity, motivation, reaction, and intuition. The subtle body connects the physical body to the brain, a connection that allows us to tune into the actions we take and the decisions we make. A yoga practice is literally a 'practice' of establishing and strengthening the connection between mind and body.

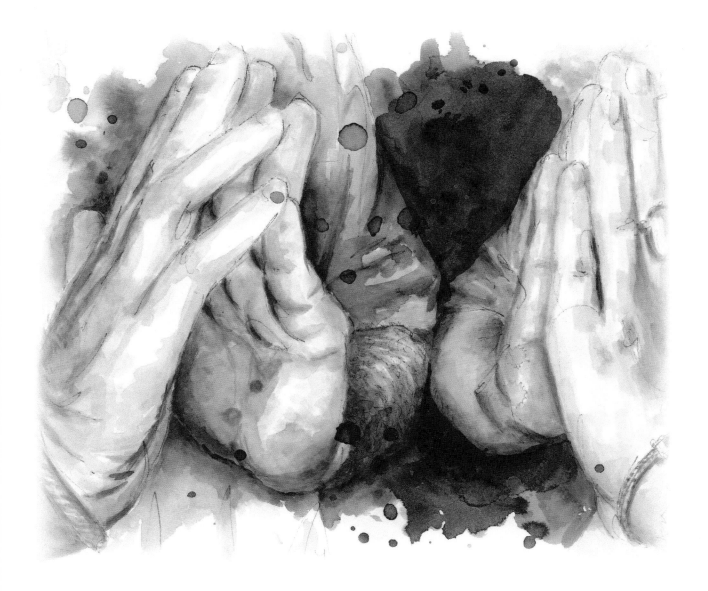

WHY MOVE FEEL THINK ?

On the yoga mat, we learn to **MOVE** the physical body by consciously placing it in different yoga poses. Next, we begin to **FEEL** each pose and experience the emotions and sensations that arise when the physical body is aligned in a certain way and engaging different energy centers. Ultimately, as the connection between body and brain grows stronger, we are able to **THINK** and process with more clarity. Our yoga practice then becomes an application of how to connect the brain and body — both on and off the mat.

A routine yoga practice can help any individual establish awareness, regain a sense of identity and purpose — and, perhaps, encourage the acceptance of lifelong changes due to brain injury, PTSD, and other forms of trauma.

13

WHY HE PRACTICES

I SUFFERED A SEVERE TRAUMATIC BRAIN INJURY IN 1996. My injuries are to the frontal lobe, which makes it difficult for me to make good decisions and interact appropriately with others. I also have trouble with self-awareness. I think part of having a brain injury is your mind disconnecting from your body, but that is hard to figure out how to fix.

I have a basic routine yoga practice with my daughter. I do things haphazardly because of my brain injury, and I learned that you cannot do yoga that way. Yoga is a discipline. You have to do the poses a certain way, and what you are doing is tying your brain to your body. They really start to interconnect, whereas on a treadmill you can turn off your brain and watch the news or listen to music. Or if you do a puzzle, you are just sitting in a chair. Yoga is physical, but it makes me think, constantly.

My wife says that yoga gets me to focus and to pay more attention to my surroundings. She says that I am less impulsive, which is a good thing. For me, it is hard to explain how exactly yoga makes me feel better. Physically it makes me walk better and have good posture, but it also helps me be normal. I got away from being normal, way off track. The yoga gets my mind and body to talk back and forth. It helps me exercise my brain, and I think that's a good thing.

Yoga can help other people with injuries like mine, but it is hard to go to a yoga class if you have a brain injury. If yoga became recognized as a treatment or a therapy, then more people with injuries to the brain could participate. I hope that we can make that happen.

John Leyde
the father.
the student.

14

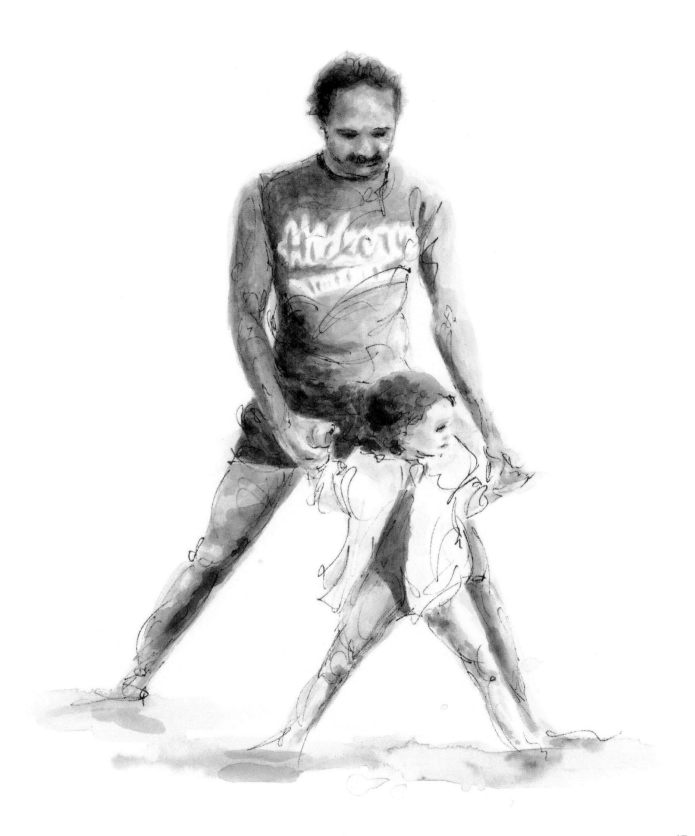

THE MOVE ‸ FEEL ⸱ THINK ‸ SEQUENCE

The **Move Feel Think** sequence can be practiced as part of a daily routine, every other day, once a week—or as often as time allows. You can take your time or move a little faster. **The most important part of this practice is to do all 20 poses in sequence.**

THE POSES

Each *vinyasa* sequence includes the following six types of poses or *asanas* (in this book, consider *asana* and pose to be one in the same): **Forward Fold, Backbend, Twist, Standing Pose, Leg Balancing Pose, Inversion.** These six types of *asana* guide the physical body across the three anatomical (or cardinal) planes.

Sagittal: front-to-back movement; flexion and extension
Coronal: side-to-side movement; abduction and adduction
Transverse rotational movement; internal rotation and external rotation

Most of us live life on the sagittal plane — walking, driving, sitting, cooking, giving someone a hug. Imagine sitting at your desk and reaching across your computer to pick up your cup of coffee — which happens to be on the left side — with your right hand. You've just moved across the transverse plane, but if you're anything like me, you probably have coffee all over your lap. That is one of reasons I love yoga. Moving and breathing and thinking on our mats is our personal opportunity to ask the body to move through its full range of motion and give the brain a chance to think clear and act without distraction.

THE SEQUENCE

As a *vinyasa* teacher, each sequence that I teach (or practice) flows through a series that includes those six types of *asana* that take the mind and body on a journey from Warm Up to Cool Down.

The **Warm Up** poses are easy movements designed to move major joints and increase blood flow to the muscles. Nothing moves too fast or makes you think too much. Here the poses stimulate the nervous and endocrine systems to prepare the body for potentially higher physical demands.

The **Standing Series** takes the practice to the next level. Having 'warmed up,' it is now time for poses that require more balance, concentration, patience, and physical strength. These poses create *tapas* (sanskrit translation: heat), which is the energy derived from each pose that we can use to wake up the body and mind.

The **Peak Pose** joins together all of the elements of the Warm Up and the Standing Series. The muscles, joints, ligaments, and brain are ready to practice trying something that might feel invigorating, unusual, uncomfortable, or just plain difficult. Think of it as breaking through.

The **Cool Down** poses are restorative. Pace and effort decrease, and the body is able to come back to baseline in restorative *asanas* that slow the heart rate and allow the muscles to relax. Now you are prepared for final rest, or *Savasana.*

THE MOVE • FEEL • THINK BENEFITS

Yoga is a practice that goes beyond the mat — beyond the physical. The practice creeps off the mat and into our conversations, actions, decisions, and relationships. This 20-pose sequence will help establish healthy relationships with the physical body as well as with others and the outside world.

MOVE

Many people are aware of the physical benefits of a yoga practice, which include everything from relieving back pain to strengthening and lengthening muscles for increased mobility. We want to sit and stand without pain, jog without strenuous effort — or even just touch our toes. "I can't do yoga, because I can't touch my toes." If I had a dollar for every time I heard someone say that. The truth is: We all want to **move** through life with ease.

On the mat we learn to flex and fold, hold and breathe, and we get comfortable with our bodies. By consciously placing the body in these different poses (*vinyasa* means to place in a special way), we build muscles and cultivate balance to support the skeletal structure. We develop proprioception (an awareness of the body in space). Yoga also aids in digestion, increases blood flow and respiratory function, and keeps the internal organs working in tandem. Yoga will help you, if you really want to, maybe touch your toes. Or, in my father's case, tie his own shoes.

FEEL

Everyone knows that exercise makes you **feel** good. In yoga you will begin to feel the poses. Once we look past the layer of the physical body, we are able to examine our emotions and reactions. You may notice that when you are feeling anxious, your heart rate goes up (physical expression due to emotional element); when you are depressed, your body feels heavy; and when you are angry, you get a little (temperature) hot.

Now that you have the moving part down you can begin to explore the ways each pose helps you feel better, how each pose helps reduce the negative feelings. Forward folds reduce anxiety by releasing what we don't need. Backbending cultivates joy as we open the space around the heart. Strong holds in warrior poses allow us to feel a sense of purpose. When the body is in alignment, engaging different energy centers, we experience emotions and sensations by tuning into a subtle (energetic) body awareness. We are able to further strengthen the connection of mind and body.

THINK

A strong mind-body connection ultimately allows us to **think** more clearly — to think before we act, to think before we talk. When we move our body around in space, to the tune of a yoga practice, we increase brain function, cognitive processing, and organizing and decision-making skills. "Yoga gets your mind in touch with your physical being," as my father says. "You want to be aware of where you are, why you're there, and how you interact. You want to think better."

A yoga practice can help us learn, and in some cases, re-learn. We learn awareness. We learn patience. We learn motivation. We learn kindness and respect — yes, to others, but also to ourselves and our joints and bones and muscles and hearts and minds. We learn freedom and love. We learn acceptance. We learn willpower — how to do more and also do less. We learn about ourselves and about how we relate to the world around us.

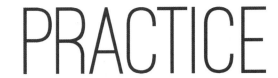

A YOGA PRACTICE TAKES DISCIPLINE.

Every person experiences trauma individually. I see brain injuries akin to snowflakes — no two injuries are identical. However, every person who lives with brain injury, PTSD, or trauma can benefit from the basic elements of a yoga practice. Yoga is personal.

Use the following tips and suggestions to help you prepare to practice the Move Feel Think sequence in this book.

First thing's first: Don't expect a darn thing. Some days you will love the poses and feel yourself growing and learning. Other days you might wish you were sitting in a traffic jam, watching paint dry, or doing the dishes. Just remember that every day is different and every practice will give you what you need on that particular day. The trick is that some days we don't know what we need. **Yoga helps us stay present. One day at a time.**

ALL YOU HAVE TO DO IS SHOW UP.

On the following pages you will find a sequence of 20 basic yoga poses—*asanas*. You can use this sequence every day, every other day, or as often as you can fit a yoga practice into your schedule.

Personally, I think 3 to 5 times a week is a good start. Depending on how often you practice, you may see positive changes in the first few weeks or months. I suggest keeping a yoga journal, where you can record what you are thinking and feeling about your practice and the poses. That way you will be able to track your thoughts and witness changes in your body over time.

THE TRUTH

The best way for trauma survivors and their caretakers to experience the positive shift that comes with a stronger mind-body connection is to practice the poses.

"DO YOUR PRACTICE
AND ALL IS COMING."

—Sri K. Pattabhi Jois

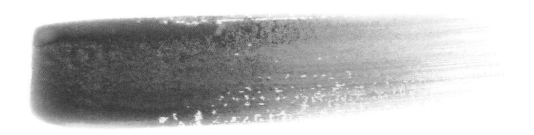

HERE'S WHAT YOU'LL NEED

TIME AND SPACE

You will need to set aside at least **30 to 45 minutes for your yoga practice**. As your practice becomes more routine, you will be able to determine the best amount of time for you. Remember — don't rush! Choose **a quiet space** to practice, and one that allows you **enough to space to roll out your mat.** (Walk all the way around the mat. If you don't bump into anything, you have enough space.) That way, if you tumble — it happens to all the best of us — you won't knock over your favorite lamp or crash into the fridge.

WHAT TO WEAR

Wear **comfortable clothes that you can move in**. If you like tight spandex, then wear that. If you like loose-fitting cotton, then wear that. But **no denim — and no shoes!**

WHAT ELSE?

SNACKS Keep some fresh water nearby — and maybe a banana (potassium) or a nutritious snack bar (protein and/or carbohydrates).

MUSIC If you like music (like me), make your favorite playlist to put on while you practice. Anything goes—meditative sounds, rock n' roll, your favorite indie band. It's *your* practice.

PHONE Turn. Off. Your. Phone. Part of creating a space for yourself to practice in is learning to step away from the outside world and all of its distractions (yogis call this *pratyahara*) so that you can focus the attention on you. One of my students calls class her "do not disturb space," which is coincidentally the name of a setting on most smartphones.

PROPS FOR PRACTICE

You will definitely want a yoga mat, but having a few other props is a very good idea. I've suggested some of my favorite brands to get you started, but you can buy these props from almost any store that sells general exercise equipment or online at amazon.com. Just remember: The better the quality of product, the longer your mats, straps, and blocks will last.

MAT Some people practice without a yoga mat, on a towel, or on a foam-like gym mat, but I urge you to use a traditional yoga mat. Yoga mats are designed for the practice and roll up nicely. **Manduka** makes slip-resistant yoga mats from sustainable materials, and they come in a myriad of colors and thicknesses.

BLANKET I do not see a reason to buy a yoga blanket if you have a large cotton or wool throw at home. But if you're in search of a traditional yoga blanket, like you see in studios, they are called Mexican blankets and Amazon has several options. Basically, you just need something to fold up on occasion to create a little padding.

BLOCKS I recommend two blocks, because there are some poses that benefit from the support of two blocks. Yoga blocks are made of either foam or cork. Foam blocks have a little bit more give to them, and that is what I use with my students. **Gaiam** makes recycled foam blocks, which come in sets of two.

STRAP There are quite a few contraption-like options out there, but I find keeping it simple is best when it comes to straps: about 1.5" x 8" long, cotton with a double D ring. If you're over six-foot, go for a 10" strap. **Yogaaccessories.com** has the most strap selections.

ADDITIONAL PROPS TO CONSIDER:

TENNIS BALLS for rolling out the feet, hands, and muscles

BOLSTERS to add a little extra in restorative, relaxing poses

MAT-SIZED MICROFIBER YOGA TOWELS if you want more grip

THE WARM UP SERIES

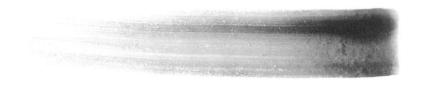

"AND YOU?
WHEN WILL YOU BEGIN
THAT LONG JOURNEY
INTO YOURSELF?"

—Rumi

1 TADASANA
MOUNTAIN POSE

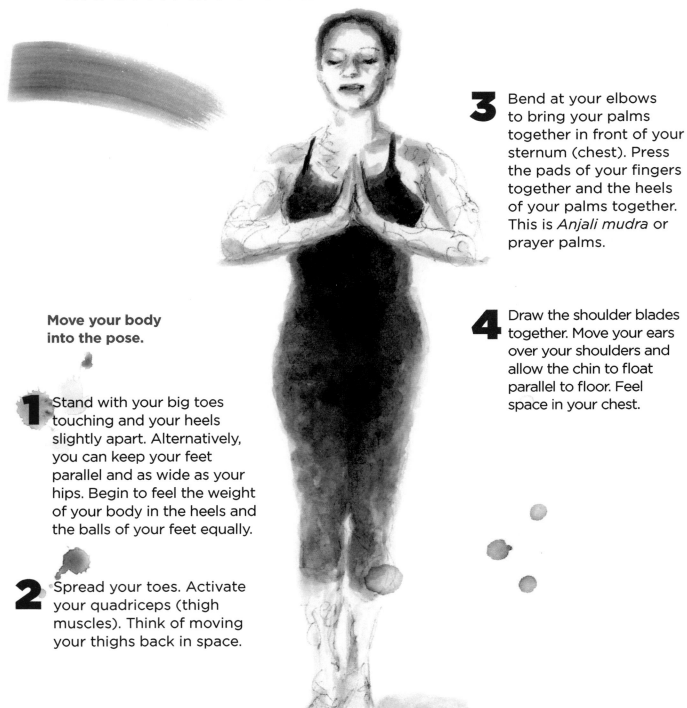

3 Bend at your elbows to bring your palms together in front of your sternum (chest). Press the pads of your fingers together and the heels of your palms together. This is *Anjali mudra* or prayer palms.

Move your body into the pose.

4 Draw the shoulder blades together. Move your ears over your shoulders and allow the chin to float parallel to floor. Feel space in your chest.

1 Stand with your big toes touching and your heels slightly apart. Alternatively, you can keep your feet parallel and as wide as your hips. Begin to feel the weight of your body in the heels and the balls of your feet equally.

2 Spread your toes. Activate your quadriceps (thigh muscles). Think of moving your thighs back in space.

HOW TO PRACTICE

Take FIVE breaths.

Feel the length of your body all the way from your feet to the top of your head. It makes no difference if you sway a little or stand steady. Allow this pose to show you where you are in the present moment.

EXTRA: Close your eyes. Maybe you will lift an inch taller.

PROP: Place a block between your inner, upper thighs. Hug the block with the muscles of your inner thighs to active the legs.

THE BENEFITS

- tones ankles, thighs, abdomen, and glutes
- reduces flat feet
- improves posture

FEEL
- cultivates self-awareness
- grounds and centers
- increases mindfulness

- improves concentration
- develops proprioception and spatial awareness
- increases impulse control

2 URDHVA HASTASANA

HANDS UP POSE

Move your body into the pose from *Tadasana*.

1 Lift both of your arms overhead, palms facing each other, arms shoulder-width apart.

2 Drop your shoulders away from your ears as you reach your fingertips high to the sky.

3 Bring your tailbone toward your heels, which aligns your pelvis and takes the curve out of your lower back. Gaze straight forward or up between your hands

4 Ground down through both feet. Think about how much space you can create between your hands and feet.

HOW TO PRACTICE

Take FIVE breaths.

Feel the weight in the balls and heels of your feet, keeping you connected to the earth. As your arms lift up, let your shoulders drop down your back so you are not holding tension.

EXTRA: Bring your prayer palms together overhead and look up at your hands. Lift your chest.

PROP: Place a block between your palms and press your palms into the block. You should feel every muscle in your arms working.

THE BENEFITS

MOVE
- opens shoulders and chest
- reduces fatigue
- improves digestion

FEEL
- relieves anxiety
- improves self-confidence
- increases initiative

THINK
- improves communication
- calms the mind
- increases self-discipline

3 UTTANASANA
FORWARD FOLD

Move your body into the pose from *Urdhva Hastasana*.

1 Lift your fingertips to the sky and ground down through your feet. This will lengthen your spine.

2 On an exhale, bend your knees slightly — bend your knees a lot if you have tight hamstrings. Hinge at your hips to fold forward and let the arms drop down to your mat. Don't worry if you can't touch the floor. That doesn't matter.

3 Draw your navel back to your spine. Think: Suck in your belly.

4 Shake your head *yes* and then *no* to release the muscles of your neck and shoulders.

HOW TO PRACTICE

Take FIVE breaths.

Release your head, letting go of any tension along the spine — all the way from your occipital ridge (the base of your brain) to your tailbone. See what happens when you sway right to left, then front to back. You can always separate the feet hip-width distance apart.

EXTRA: Grab opposite elbows. Do this by crossing your forearms and bringing the palms of each hand to the opposite elbow.

PROP: Place a block under each palm. As you press the palms into the blocks, lift your tailbone to the sky. Make sure to keep your neck loose and your knees slightly bent for tight hamstrings.

THE BENEFITS

MOVE
- stretches hamstrings, calf muscles, and hips
- stimulates kidneys and liver
- relieves headaches, high blood pressure, and sinusitis

FEEL
- relieves depression
- strenghtens sense of purpose
- increases motivation

THINK
- improves processing
- reduces mental fatigue
- increases patience

4 ARDHA UTTANASANA
HALF LIFT

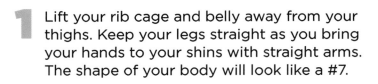

Move your body into the pose from *Uttanasana*.

1 Lift your rib cage and belly away from your thighs. Keep your legs straight as you bring your hands to your shins with straight arms. The shape of your body will look like a #7.

2 Extend the back of your neck. You can do this by looking at a space on the floor beyond your toes.

3 Draw your navel back to your spine. By engaging the abdominals, you support the back.

4 Bring the bottom tips of your shoulder blades together. Feel your chest start to broaden and the sides of your body get longer.

HOW TO PRACTICE

Take FIVE breaths.

Press your hands into your shins. Press your heels into the floor and spread your toes. Picture one long line of energy flowing all the way from your tailbone to the crown of your head.

EXTRA: Keep your back as is, but bring your hands to your hips. Let your elbows wing out to the sides as you stay engaged through the abdominals. Keep a micro-bend (very small) in your knees.

PROP: Place a block between your inner, upper thighs. Hug the block with your upper thighs as you bring the body into the #7 shape of this pose.

THE BENEFITS

MOVE
- strengthens back and the lower abdominals
- relieves insomnia, asthma, and headaches
- lowers blood pressure

FEEL
- reduces anxiety
- lessens fear of change
- increases intuition, or sense of Self

THINK
- reduces judgment
- improves decision-making skills
- decreases fixation

VINYASA FLOW
THREE SUN BREATHS

Once you have practiced poses 1-4. You can create a *vinyasa* flow by doing those four poses in a sequence called a **Sun Breath.** Try to initiate the breath before the movement for each pose. This will help you link body to brain. You can do **Sun Breaths** first thing in the morning or anytime during the day when you might need a little movement, a little balance, or a little something to calm you down.

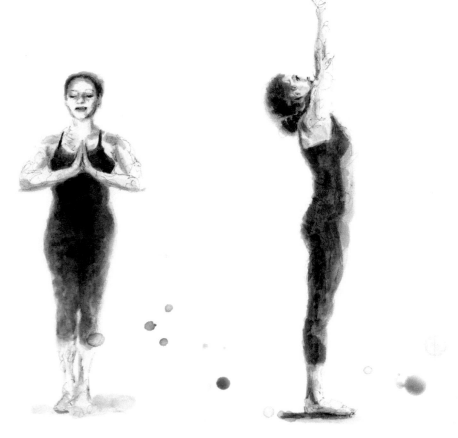

1

Start by standing in *Tadasana.*

2 INHALE

Lift your arms wide to the side and overhead for *Urdhva Hastasana,* Hands Up Pose.

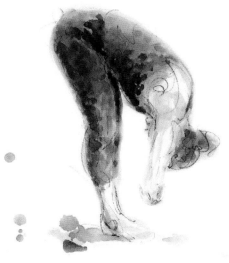

3 EXHALE

Fold over to
Uttanasana,
Forward Fold.

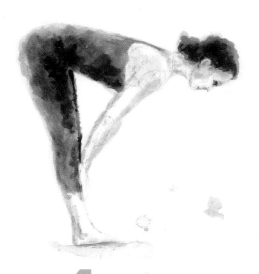

4 INHALE

Lift to a flat back,
Ardha Uttanasana.

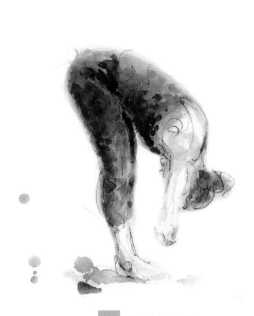

5 EXHALE

Fold over,
Uttanasana.

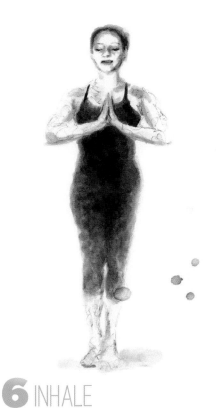

6 INHALE

Roll one vertebra at a
time all the way back
up to *Tadasana.*

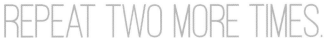
REPEAT TWO MORE TIMES.

THE FIRST LIMB OF YOGA

THE FIVE YAMAS

PRACTICE OUTER OBSERVANCE: BE GOOD TO OTHERS.

The *yamas* are our attitudes and behaviors toward other people and our environment.

AHIMSA **Non-violence:** Show compassion toward all living things. Do not harm yourself or others. Be kind. Be kind to animals, to your environment, to your family and friends, even to strangers. Be kind to yourself — always. Eat well. Wave back. Smile more. Express gratitude. As my grandmother would say, "Think kind thoughts. Do good things."

What is not *ahimsa*: hurting yourself; hurting others; being mean to animals; littering

How to practice *ahimsa*: Before you do or say something, think about the other person. Think: Would I enjoy a person doing or saying this to me?

SATYA **Truthfulness:** Do not lie. Do not fib or exaggerate. Do not lie to yourself. Live what is true. Be who you are right now. *Sat* is the root word for truth. I have the Sanskrit symbol for *sat* tattooed on my right wrist, as part of the mantra *Om Tat Sat*, which, in so many words, means "All there is is truth." It reminds me to be true to myself and to others.

What is not *satya*: lying about where you were; about what you said; lying about anything; telling someone you did something that something you didn't do; telling yourself or someone else that something is okay when it is not okay

How to practice *satya*: Speak the truth. Even when it might be easier to lie, see how you can communicate with honesty.

ASTEYA — **Non-stealing:** Do not take from others. Do not steal. Do not take what is not freely given. Do not demand things of others. Do not take advantage of others. Say "thank you" for the gifts you receive — big or small. Show up on time when you are meeting others for meetings or classes or parties or dinner dates.

What is not *asteya*: stealing from the store; stealing something from someone else; arriving late to meet a friend; taking anything that does not belong to you

How to practice *asteya*: Appreciate all of things you have. Before you go to sleep at night, make a mental list of the things you are grateful for and you will focus less on what others have that you may not.

BRAHMACHARYA — **Self-restraint:** Do not expend energy on things that do not serve a purpose. Gain control over your impulses. Do not live in excess or be wasteful. Invest your time, efforts, and resources wisely. "All things in moderation," which is the best advice I have ever received, which came from my mother.

What is not *brahmacharya*: fixating on getting a new car; fixating on getting a particular job; fixating on what you cannot have; fixating on anything.

How to practice *brahmacharya*: Choose purposeful thoughts and actions. Direct them toward a goal that leads to more happiness and a greater sense of purpose.

APARIGRAHA — **Non-seizing:** Let go of what you do not need. Do not compare what you do not have to what others have. Do not be jealous. Know the difference between *need* and *want*. As my father often says, "You don't ever get what you want, because then you don't want it anymore." Kind of true, Dad.

What is not *aparigraha*: eating the entire cake or the whole bag of pretzels; leaving the lights and the TV on when you leave; being greedy; coveting

How to practice *aparigraha*: Become aware of what you consume. Conserve energy. Share what you have. Let go.

THE SECOND LIMB OF YOGA

THE FIVE NIYAMAS

PRACTICE INNER OBSERVANCE: BE GOOD TO YOU.

The *niyamas* are our attitudes and behaviors toward ourselves, how we treat our mind and body.

SAUCHA   **Cleanliness:** Maintain a clean body, inside and out. Practice personal hygiene. Eat foods that nourish the body. Maintain a clean environment — your home, your car, your room, your kitchen. Maintain a clean mind. Release any disturbing emotions, such as fear, anger, hate, lust, delusion, and want.

What is not *saucha*: not cleaning up after yourself; not washing your body or your clothes; eating junk food for dinner

How to practice *saucha*: After yoga practice, wipe down your mat and roll it up nicely. Put away the other props you use. Pick up after yourself.

SANTOSA   **Contentment:** Be at peace with the present. Aspire toward acceptance. It is the mantra of *Om Tat Sat* ("All that is is truth.") Do not continuously grieve or complain about your present state, but learn from it. By living as best as we can in present conditions, we are able to cultivate hopefulness.

What is not *santosa*: not accepting change; demanding that you are same the person you always have been; refusing to move on from difficult circumstances

How to practice *santosa*: Get to know the person you are after a traumatic experience. Acknowledge the changes. Learn from that person.

TAPAS   **Self-Discipline:** Find a disciplined use for your energy — your heat, your fire, your will. Stay active. Stay motivated. Keep the physical body in shape by burning energy, exercising, and eating well. Exercise your will power.

What is not *tapas:* sleeping past noon; watching TV all day long; never leaving your house; complaining

How to practice *tapas:* Do yoga. A yoga practice not only draws attention to the physical body but also creates good posture, healthy eating habits, regular breathing patterns, and a clear mind.

SVADHYAYA   **Study of self:** Get to know yourself. Practice self-awareness. Through self-inquiry we learn our patterns, weaknesses, and addictions. We also learn what illuminates our soul. Pick a hobby — write, draw, paddleboard, play chess, play the violin, walk dogs, ride horses, volunteer, bake pies — and stick with it. This practice will help you uncover your strengths and accept your limitations.

What is not *svadhyaya:* comparing yourself to other people; fueling addictions; refusing to get help when you could use some

How to practice *svadhyaya:* Get to know yourself on the mat. Who are you in that space? What enlivens you? What frustrates you? And how can you learn to accept and celebrate this? Take what you learn off the mat.

ISHVARA PRANIDHANA   **Devotion:** Surrender control. Release expectations. Let go. Know that life is never really going to work out that way we had it planned. Know there is a bigger picture. Find meaning. Ask yourself how you can serve others with what you are capable of.

What is not *ishvara pranidhana:* trying to control what you cannot control; resisting change; fighting reality

How to practice *ishvara pranidhana:* Garden. Pray. Meditate. Breathe deeper. Stare at the stars. Walk on a beach. Listen to music. Stand in the rain. Do anything that celebrates something bigger, grander, and beyond your own existence.

IF THE YAMAS AND NIYAMAS DON'T MAKE SENSE OR SEEM DAUNTING, SIMPLY THINK OF THEM AS GUIDELINES TO HELP YOU BE KIND, INSIDE AND OUT.

THE STANDING SERIES

"YOGA TEACHES US
TO CURE WHAT
NEED NOT BE ENDURED
AND ENDURE WHAT
CANNOT BE CURED."

—B.K.S. Iyengar

5 VIRABHADRASANA I
WARRIOR ONE

Move your body into the pose from *Tadasana*.

1 Step your left foot back behind you — at least 3 feet.

2 Place your hands on your hips and angle your left foot so that the toes are pointing to upper left corner of your mat. If you feel like it's hard to balance, move your right foot to the right a few inches. Think: two feet on railroad tracks, not on a tightrope.

3 Bend your right knee, allowing your thigh to come closer to parallel to the floor. Look down and make sure you can see your toes in front of your knee. You do not want your knee beyond your ankle. Ouch.

4 Reach both arms overhead—like in *Urdhva Hastasana.*

40

HOW TO PRACTICE

Take FIVE breaths.

Press the big toe of your right foot into the floor and the outer edge of your left foot into the floor. Feel energy and strength in both legs.

EXTRA: Hook your right thumb into your right hip crease. Pull back and down. Take your left palm around your outer left hip and press forward. These two actions align the hips to face forward, which will get you deeper into the pose.

PROP: Place a block between your hands and press your palms into the block. Drop your shoulders. Now your arms are working.

TWO SIDES: Step forward to *Tadasana*. Step the right foot back and repeat on the other side for another FIVE breaths.

THE BENEFITS

MOVE
- opens hips and chest
- improves balance
- relieves sciatica

FEEL
- builds self-confidence
- increases motivation
- strengthens intuition

THINK
- improves memory
- reduces fixation
- increases understanding

6 VIRABHADRASANA II
WARRIOR TWO

Move your body into the pose from *Tadasana*.

1 Step your left foot back behind you—at least 3 to 4 feet.

2 Place your hands on your hips and angle your left foot so that the toes are pointing directly to the left. Look down to see the heel of your front foot intersecting the arch of your back foot. If this is too narrow to balance, move your right foot to the right a few inches.

4 Reach your arms out to the side, like a T, palms face down. Extend your fingertips away from each other. Turn your entire upper body to face the left.

3 Bend your right knee, allowing the thigh to come closer to parallel to the floor. Look down and make sure you can see your toes in front of your knee. You do not want your knee beyond your ankle. Ouch. This will feel a little different from *Virabhadrasana I*, especially in your hips and back leg.

HOW TO PRACTICE

Take FIVE breaths.

Move your inner front knee away from center so the knee aligns over the ankle. Ground down through the outer edge of your back foot. Feel energy and strength in both legs.

EXTRA: Inhale. Lift your arms over your head. Exhale. Extend the arms back out to the sides. Repeat 4 more times, inhaling to lift and exhaling to extend.

TWO SIDES: Step forward to *Tadasana*. Step your right foot back and repeat on the other side for another FIVE breaths.

THE BENEFITS

 MOVE
- opens hips
- stimulates abdominal organs
- alleviates flat feet, carpal tunnel syndrome, and back pain

 FEEL
- builds stamina
- grounds and centers
- increases independence

 THINK
- improves organization and planning
- increases concentration
- calms the mind

7 PRASARITA PADOTTANASANA
WIDE-LEGGED FORWARD FOLD

How to move your body into the pose from *Virabhadrasana II—on the left side:*

1 Bring your hands to your hips. Pivot on your heels so that all ten toes are facing right. Extend your arms out to the sides. See that your feet are parallel to the edges of your mat — and as wide as your outstretched arms.

2 Press into the outer edges of each foot, like you are pushing the feet away from one another. Keep a slight bend in the knees.

3 Hug your inner thighs together. Pressing out, hugging in — opposing actions for the muscles, but your legs don't really move.

4 Hinge forward at your hips and allow your arms and hands to fall to floor as you lower into a wide-legged forward fold. Let your hands, arms, back, and neck hang loose, a little like *Uttanasana*.

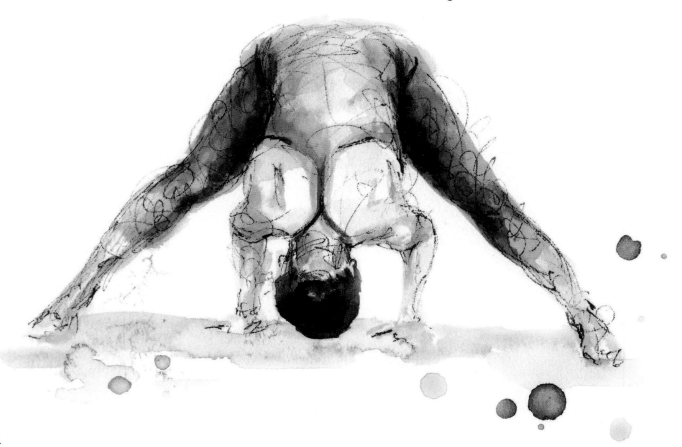

HOW TO PRACTICE

Take FIVE breaths.

Bring the weight into the balls of your feet. Draw your navel back to your spine. Know that feeling lightheaded is absolutely normal when the head goes below the heart. If you feel like you might tip over, your hands are on the mat and they will catch you. If you feel dizzy when you come up, come up slower. If you feel too dizzy, don't go down so low.

EXTRA: As you stay strong and activate through your legs, allow your head to bobble. Close your eyes and imagine the crown of your head dripping toward the floor. Let go of every thought or feeling you don't need.

PROP: Place a block underneath the bridge of your nose. Bring your chin to your chest and rest the crown of your head (the top) on top of the block. You can use the block at any height to make that connection. If you need a little extra, place a fist (or two) on top of the block and rest the top of your head on your fist.

THE BENEFITS

MOVE
- lengthens spine
- reduces fatigue
- strengthens inner thighs and back of legs

FEEL
- increases sympathy and compassion
- creates feeling of abundance
- grounds and centers

THINK
- improves reasoning
- increases processing
- calms the parasympathetic nervous system

8 TRIKONASANA
TRIANGLE POSE

How to move your body into the pose from *Prasarita Padottanasana:*

1 Bring your hands to your hips. Use the strength of your abdominals to lift up to a flat back and all the way up to stand tall.

2 Pivot your right heel so the toes face the upper right corner of the mat. Pivot your left heel so that the toes face the top of your mat. A little like *Virabhadrasana I* feet, but with a straight front leg.

3 Extend your arms straight out to the sides—like a T. The chest faces the right. Just like in *Virabhadrasana II.*

4 Reach the left hand down to the left shin. Extend the right hand up to the sky. If it's comfortable for your neck, turn your head to look up to the right fingertips.

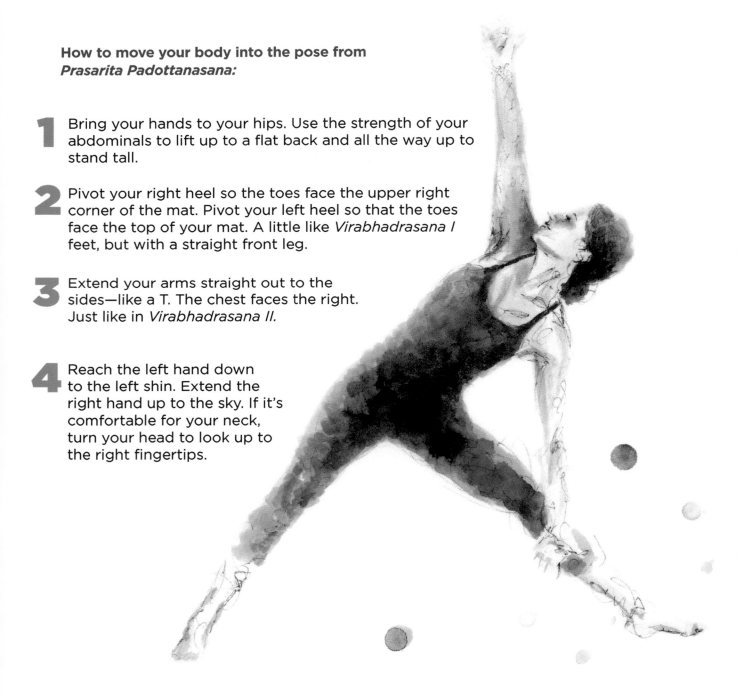

HOW TO PRACTICE

Take FIVE breaths.

Press down through both feet. Begin to rotate the left side of your ribs over to the right, opening your heart. Feel your hips open, while your right shoulder starts to stack on top of the left.

EXTRA: Extend your top arm over your ear and reach the fingertips toward the front of your mat. Be careful not to smash your arm into your face, so drop the right shoulder blade down your spine. This is call *Utthita Trikonasana*, which is "extended triangle pose."

PROP: Place a block on either side of the front foot. Press down into the block with your left hand to get more lift through the pose as you continue to reach the opposite arm overhead. Spin your chest upward.

TWO SIDES: Press into your feet and lift up to stand. Pivot on both heels so all ten toes are facing right. Repeat on the other side for another FIVE breaths—you will face the back of your mat for this side. Then step forward to *Tadasana,* back to the front of your mat.

THE BENEFITS

MOVE
- tones back, neck, and abdominals
- stretches hips and groin
- increases metabolism and improves digestion

FEEL
- reduces stress and anxiety
- increases empathy
- improves self-awareness

THINK
- improves communication
- increases attention span
- clears the mind

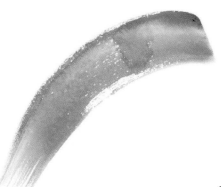

9 VRKSASANA
TREE POSE

How to move your body into the pose from *Tadasana:*

1 Bring your hands to *Anjali mudra,* prayer palms. Begin to transfer the weight into your left foot. Come onto the ball of your right foot. For more balance, bring your hands to your hips.

2 Choose one point of focus to send a soft gaze — a *drishti.* Choose something that is in front of you and not moving.

3 Lift up your right knee to hip level. Start to let the right knee open out to the side, like you are swinging a door open gently.

4 Place the sole of your right foot on your inner ankle, inner calf, or inner thigh — anywhere but your knee. You can use the right hand to help you adjust, but make sure you are placing the foot in a place that still allows you to stand tall with a straight spine and open heart. Come back to your *drishti.*

HOW TO PRACTICE

Take FIVE breaths.

Press your prayer palms together and feel your collarbones get wide. Try not to grip the mat with your toes or clench your jaw. Don't worry if your tree topples. Maybe try lifting your arms overhead. Send your breath to your balance, your mind to your drishti.

EXTRA: Try it with your eyes closed!

TWO SIDES: Drop your right foot back down to *Tadasana* — take your time. Take a breath or two standing on two feet. Begin *Vrksasana* on the opposite side for FIVE breathes.

THE BENEFITS

MOVE
- strengthens legs and pelvis
- improves posture
- relieves sciatica

FEEL
- boosts self-esteem
- fosters emotional balance
- creates a sense of calm

THINK
- develops proprioception and spatial awareness
- improves balance and coordination
- increases concentration

10 UTKATASANA
AWKWARD CHAIR POSE

How to move your body into the pose from *Tadasana*:

1 Lift your arms overhead — like *Urdhva Hastasana* arms. Bend your knees and sit your hips back and down, like you are sitting into a chair.

2 Draw your belly back to your spine. Think: Sit back to sit low.

3 Look down to see if you can see your toes. See that your knees are in line with one another, which will tell you what your hips are doing.

4 Squeeze your inner, upper thighs together. Draw the bottom tips of your shoulder blades together.

HOW TO PRACTICE

Take FIVE breaths.

Continue to sit back to sit low. Drop your tailbone to your heels to feel a little more space in your lower back. Lift the chest (but don't crunch the neck) to look up to the space between your palms. Feel your spine long. To come out of the pose, fold over bent legs into *Uttanasana.* Then roll back up to stand in *Tadasana.*

EXTRA: Bring your palms to heart center, *Anjali mudra.* Begin to twist over to the right side. See if you can hook your left elbow on the outside of your right thigh — *Parivrtta Utkatasana*, Revolved Chair Pose. Keep squeezing the knees and inner thighs. Maybe look up to the ceiling as the chest rotates to the right. Try the other side.

PROP: Place a block near the top of your mat on the lowest height. Step just your heels on the block, toes on the mat (it will look like you are wearing high heels). Sit back into Chair Pose over the block. Squeeze your ankles, calves, and thighs together. By balancing on a block, you automatically draw your energy in toward your midline, strengthening the pose and toning the inner thighs — a lot! Plus, it's good for balance.

THE BENEFITS

MOVE
- opens chest and shoulders
- stimulates diaphragm and heart
- strengthens hip flexors

FEEL
- stabilizes mood and emotions
- lessens feelings of apathy
- relieves depression

THINK
- improves impulse control
- increases focus and attention span
- strengthens balance

VINYASA FLOW STANDING POSES

Once you have practiced poses 5-10, you can create a **Vinyasa flow** by doing these six poses in a sequence. You can also add these on to **Sun Breaths**. Even though the *asanas* may be trickier, try to initiate the breath before the movement in each pose, which will help strengthen that connection of body to brain. If you need a break, take a pause for a few breaths in *Tadasana* or *Uttanasana*.

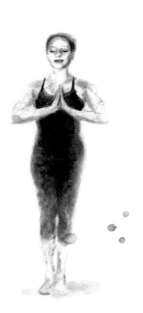

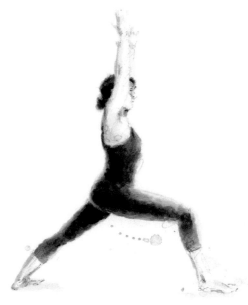

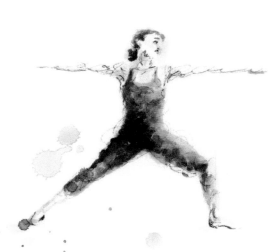

1
Start by standing in *Tadasana.*

2 INHALE
Step your left foot back to *Virabhadrasana I.*

EXHALE

3 INHALE
Pivot on your back heel so toes face the side to find your *Virabhadrasana II*.

EXHALE

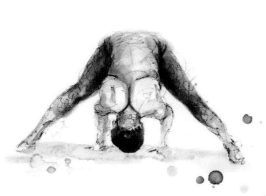

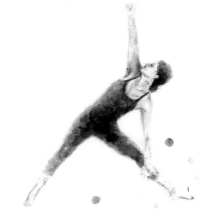

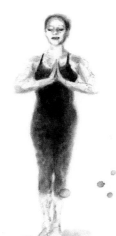

4 INHALE

Straighten both legs, pivot on your heels, and find yourself in **Prasarita Padottanasana,** wide-legged forward fold.

EXHALE

5 INHALE

Roll up to stand. Stretch your arms out to a T. Pivot your right heel so the toes face the top of your mat. Reach your right arm forward and lower to the calf or ankle for **Trikonasana,** Triangle Pose.

EXHALE

6 INHALE

Rise up and step your left foot forward to **Tadasana.**

EXHALE

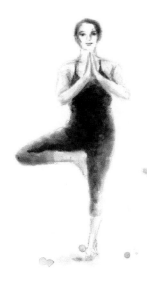

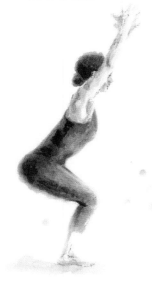

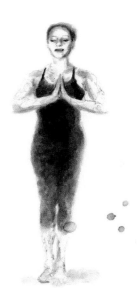

7 INHALE

Lift your right foot into **Vrksasana.** Hold for 3 breaths. Exhale to *Tadasana.*

8 INHALE

Sit back over your heels for chair pose, **Utkatasana,** Awkward Chair.

EXHALE

9 INHALE

Tadasana.

Repeat sequence on the left side by stepping the right foot back for *Virabhadrasana I.*

THE THIRD LIMB OF YOGA

ASANA

PRACTICE THE PHYSICAL POSES:
ASANA MEANS POSTURE.

This physical practice keeps the body healthy and in harmony with nature.

When most of us think of yoga, we think of the *asana* practice. *Asana* is the reason we roll out our mats — to bend, flex, strengthen, and lengthen the body. *Asana* is what keeps us fit. It burns those *tapas.* It is physical exercise. However, if we're talking about the yogic path, *asana* is only one limb out of eight. *Asana* follows the *yamas* and the *niyamas,* because once we are able to understand how we exist, react, and contribute to our outer and inner worlds, we are able to step onto the mat and get to know the physical body through an *asana* practice.

"The posture of yoga is steady and easy," said Pantanjali, a yoga sage said to have composed *The Yoga Sutras,* a classical yoga text made up of 195 aphorisms that we teachers often turn to for nuggets of wisdom. Yoga postures are a balance of *sthira* (strength, steadiness) and *sukha* (joy, ease). Although the *asanas* are mostly physical exercises filled with movement, these postures (and there are thousands) were designed to prepare the body to sit comfortably in stillness, just like those happy, tubby, cross-legged Buddhas who are sitting in what's called *Sukhasana* (Easy Pose).

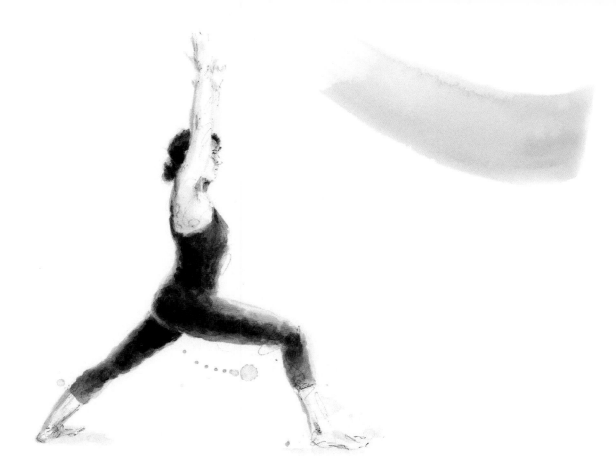

When I begin my classes, nine times out of ten, I will start seated. I either sit up on a block or blanket, with one shin folded in front of the other, as I give my message to my students. I'm sitting in *Sukhasana*, and it's never "easy" for me. I was one of those kids in elementary school who could not sit Indian style. Every time I tried to sit that way, like the other kids and the Native Americans and the Buddhas, my hips hurt, my feet fell asleep, and my back ached. Eventually I gave up. It was just never comfortable, not even as a kid.

Today, after years and years of moving, breathing, twisting, flexing, and bending with my *asana* practice, Easy Pose comes with a little more ease. I may never be able to fold my legs on top of one another in *Padmasana* (Lotus Pose), and my knees may never flop down flush with the floor, but I have created more space in my hips, strength in my back, and patience for the sensations that arise. I am learning to be still as an adult.

Still, where there is no reaction to the tweaks and tickles, to the thoughts and distractions. It's a stillness that can be found in five breaths of *Virabhadrasana I* or in five minutes of meditation. In stillness — between *sthira* and *sukha* — the mind is calm. In stillness we find the rhythm of breath which helps us to connect brain and body.

THE FOURTH LIMB OF YOGA

PRANAYAMA

PRACTICE THE RHYTHMIC CONTROL OF BREATH: PRANA MEANS LIFE FORCE, BREATH, OR VITAL ENERGY.

This practice fills the body with *prana* to clear the mind and cultivate mindfulness.

Think of the *asana* practice as what clears out space in the body. With no space in the physical body, there is no room for breath or *prana*. Our state of mind is closely linked to the quality of *prana* within. Someone who lacks *prana* is troubled, confused, restless, or physically unwell. Too little *prana* also leads to feelings of frustration, depression, and apathy.

Filling the body with *prana* starts with controlling the pattern of breath through inhales and exhales. We move through our days giving little thought to our breath. We rarely put breath first, because it will always be there — even at the last minute. A yoga practice gives us the opportunity to put the breath first. I often tell my students to "initiate breath before movement," a line I use from one of my friends and favorite teachers. This is one of the simplest ways to connect breath to body, and it is the breath that tethers brain to body.

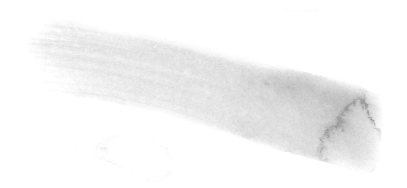

When you establish a control of breath, it will eventually lead to a smoother physical practice. Certain poses will come with more ease as you learn to inhale *prana* and send that life force to any tricky or tight spots in the physical body. Over time, your practice will begin to open up from the inside out. Eventually, you can dive into the umpteen different *pranayama* exercises that come with a more advanced yoga practice. The most commonly practiced *pranayama* is *Ujjayi* (Victorious Breath). It is the slight constriction of the throat as you inhale and exhale out through the nose, which is the same sensation of talking in a whisper or fogging up a window. This breath makes the sound of ocean waves rolling in and out. *Ujjayi* calms the body, especially in complicated or challenging postures or situations. *Ujjayi* can also energize the body when you are feeling fatigued.

There is also *Simhasana* (Lion's Breath) to surrender control. *Kapalabhati* (Breath of Fire) is the Ego Eradicator; its short, rapid exhales help shine the skull — or clear the mind. *Brahmari* (Bee Breath) is practiced by making a humming sound while closing the eyes and plugging the ears to shut off the world; it helps with anxiety. And *Nadi Shodhana,* (Alternate Nostril Breathing) synchronizes the hemispheres of the brain and brings the body in balance.

Linking *asana* and *pranayama* is the path to linking brain and body. Soon you will be able to take this calmness cultivated by breath off the yoga mat into real life. Breath helps the body to *move* with more ease, and it helps the mind to *be* more at ease in stillness.

THE
PEAK POSE

"TO PERFORM EVERY ACTION ARTFULLY IS YOGA."

—Swami Kripalu

11 MARJARYASANA/BITILASANA
CAT/COW POSE

How to move your body into the pose from *Tadasana*:

1 Bend your knees a lot, so much so that you can place your hands on the mat. Step your feet back, drop your knees, and come to all fours. If you have sensitive knees put a blanket underneath your knees.

2 Place your hands underneath your shoulders, and spread your fingers wide — like a starfish.

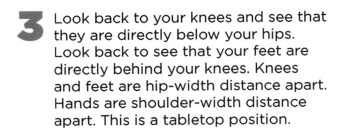

3 Look back to your knees and see that they are directly below your hips. Look back to see that your feet are directly behind your knees. Knees and feet are hip-width distance apart. Hands are shoulder-width distance apart. This is a tabletop position.

4 Press the tops of the feet, all ten toenails, your shins, and your hands into the mat. Engage your lower belly for a strong, flat back.

HOW TO PRACTICE

Take FIVE Cat/Cow undulations — FIVE breaths.

Inhale. Lift your sternum and bring your chest forward. Look up. Allow your tailbone to lift up as your belly drops down. This is COW. The center of your back is dipping down.

Exhale. Draw your belly back to your spine. Arch your back and allow the crown of your head to drop toward the floor. This is CAT. The center of your back is rounding up.

EXTRA: As you lift into Cow, bend your elbows and sway over to one side. As you lift up for Cat, bend your knees and sway to the opposite side. Using these movements, start to draw circular-like movements with your body. One half of the circle is the inhale and the other half is the exhale. It doesn't have to be perfect.

PROP: Place a block long-ways between your inner upper thighs. Squeeze the block as you move through Cat/Cow. The block will stabilize your hips.

THE BENEFITS

MOVE
- strengthens and stretches abdominals
- increases mobility of the spine
- stimulates adrenal glands and kidneys

FEEL
- creates emotional balance
- increases self-confidence
- overcomes fear

THINK
- reduces judgment
- improves coordination
- strengthens understanding

12 ADHO MUKHA SVANASANA
DOWNWARD FACING DOG

How to move your body into the pose from Cat/Cow:

1 Tuck your toes under and come up on the balls of your feet. Press into both hands equally and begin to lift your knees off the mat. This might be difficult. Go at your own pace. Remember not to hold your breath.

2 Lift the hips up to sky. Stay strong through your arms and hands as your legs begin to get a little straighter and more weight goes into your feet.

3 Press your thighs back in space. If you have tight hamstrings, keep your knees bent. You can always keep your knees slightly bent in Downward Dog.

4 Lift your belly and your rib cage away from the mat. Round your tailbone to your heels — it's a little like a Cat Pose back. You want to feel length in the spine, strength in the belly, and openness in the chest.

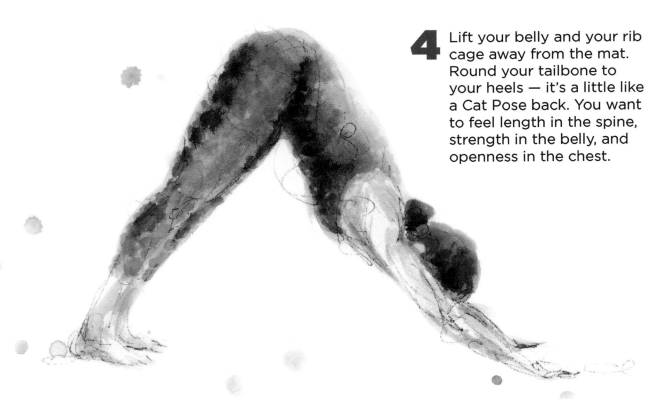

HOW TO PRACTICE

Take FIVE breaths.

Spread your fingers wide like in Cat/Cow. Press down into your thumb and the knuckle joint at the base of your index finger. Roll your upper arms away from your ears. Think: Turn your armpits to your ears. Stay active through the lower half of your body by grounding down through the outer edge of each foot. Don't worry if your heels don't touch the mat. Try to find equal weight and energy between the bottom half and the top half of your body.

EXTRA: Inhale. Lift your right leg back behind you. Toes face down and heel faces up. Exhale. Lower back down to Down Dog. Inhale. Lift your left leg back behind you, toes facing down, heel facing up. Exhale. Lower down to Down Dog. Imagine someone had a string attached to your heel and was pulling it straight up to the ceiling. Try this two more times.

PROP: Place a block on the lowest height underneath each palm to give you a little bit more lift to help send the energy and weight into the lower half of your body.

THE BENEFITS

MOVE
- builds bone density
- increases circulation
- relieves headaches

FEEL
- boosts energy and stamina
- reduces anxiety
- releases trapped emotions

THINK
- improves processing and executive function
- increases decision-making
- calms the mind

13 BALASANA
CHILD'S POSE

Move your body into the pose from *Adho Mukha Svanasana:*

1 Walk the feet together so your toes are touching. Bend your knees and let them drop down to your mat.

2 Untuck your toes and let your hips sit back over your heels. Let your arms extend out in front of you or back by your hips. Choose whichever allows you to relax more.

3 Rest your third eye (the space between your eyebrows) on the mat. If your forehead does not reach the mat, you can slide a blanket or block underneath. You want to be able to connect it to something solid.

4 Relax every muscle in your body.

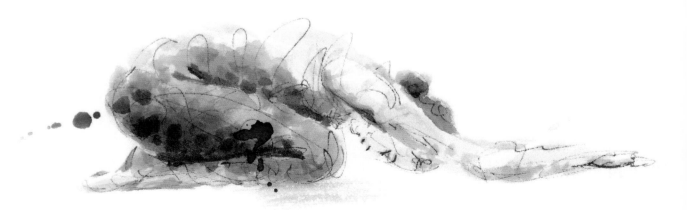

HOW TO PRACTICE

Take TEN breaths.

This is a restorative, relaxation pose. Keep your belly soft. Try not to grip with your hands or hips. Feel yourself sinking down into your mat. You can even interlace your fingers and place them, palms facing down, on the back of your head with your elbows winging out to each side for more grounding.

EXTRA: If you have tight hips, take your knees wide to the sides of your mat. Let your belly rest between your thighs and breathe into your hips. Or, if you have tension in your lower back, bring your knees together toward the center. Let your spine round and breathe into your lower back.

PROP: Fold your blanket in half and then in half again. Keep this tight bundle and place it at the back of your knee creases. Sit back down into Child's Pose.

THE BENEFITS

MOVE
- stretches hips, thighs, and ankles
- relieves back and neck pain
- reduces dizziness or fatigue

FEEL
- cultivates forgiveness
- introduces a sense of peace and tranquility
- restores emotional balance

THINK
- improves reasoning
- increases problem solving-skills
- develops understanding

THE FIFTH LIMB OF YOGA

PRATYAHARA

PRACTICE DETACHMENT:
PRATYAHARA MEANS THE WITHDRAWAL OF THE SENSES.

It is the hinge of yoga, the point of being able to shift from the outer to the inner world.

It is easy to clutter our lives with feelings and opinions. We assign thousands of adjectives — good, bad, amazing, horrific, healthy, challenging, crazy, gorgeous, important — to the actions, objects, and relationships of our everyday lives. We allow the stories we tell about things to dictate our relationship with those things. In Sanskrit this is called *Chitta-vritti*, which means mind-stuff, or mind chatter. It's our monkey mind. Sutra 1.2: *Yoga citta vritti nirodhah.* Yoga is the resolutions of the agitations of the mind.

Sit down in the middle of a Times Square sidewalk. Just plop down and cross your legs and close your eyes. Do it right smack dab among the throngs of New York City. What would you experience? Noise — lots of it. There would be sirens and traffic and buses, people talking to you, people talking to other people about you. Sensations — yes. You would feel the gushes of air from the subway grates or from the passing cars, the concrete under your skin, people's shopping bags brushing against you. And the smells — street food, steam from sewers, car exhaust, wafts of perfume. Could you sit still and not move? Could you not react?

Heck no, that'd be crazy! Scary. Weird. Impossible. Really stupid? Well, maybe. We move through life not only experiencing our senses but reacting to them. We retract from discomfort and fear. We embrace delicious tastes and sweet smells and a warm touch. As humans, we are very attached to our external environment.

Therefore we must begin to practice how to detach, how to feel less. Detachment does not make us uncaring or cruel. And detachment is not being a yogi who lives in a cave on a mountain in Nepal in the middle of nothing and no one. Detachment is being a practitioner of yoga who can separate himself or herself from a constant stream of reactions in order to quiet the mind. Believe it or not, there are people who can sit down in Times Square and just chill. They are practicing this fifth limb of yoga, *pratyahara.*

The detachment begins with stillness. I can remember when I first started to practice yoga and the teacher would lead a meditation. I dreaded this part. Whether it was before or after class didn't matter. I would set up my seat, close my eyes, connect with my breath, and then everything on earth would bother me. I would fix a fallen piece of hair or scratch the itch on my ankle. A dog would bark, and I'd turn my head toward the window. All the outside events felt like a pinball machine in my mind.

Pratyahara is nuanced, a practice of detaching that is deep and subtle. I believe we learn it on our mats first — and it takes time. The body is opened with *asana* and filled with breath through *pranayama* to calm the mind. An open body and calm mind experience less distraction. On the mat, poses are less frustrating, less boring. Off the mat the harsh comment someone made will eventually hurt less. Traffic jams will be less infuriating. Cake will be less tempting. Memories will just be memories. *Pratyahara* has helped me release expectations and find acceptance for that which I cannot control.

DHARANA

PRACTICE CONCENTRATION: DHARANA MEANS TO HOLD.

A calm, clear mind can hold attention in one direction to focus on one thing.

To practice *dharana,* one has to be fully present. It is a one-pointed focus on one activity or one object. Focus is not to be confused with fixation. A focused mind is connected to the present moment. A fixated mind is trapped in the past or holding onto an idea of the future. Fixation feels like addiction — impossible to exist without, which is the opposite of detachment.

Dharana is focus. A detached mind is clear. Yet a clear mind can still easily wander, which diverts our attention from one thing to the other, to many thoughts and feelings at once. This is human nature. It is nearly impossible to stop our thoughts or halt the processes of our brain, so our option is to choose a focus, a concentration.

Sometimes the focus is as simple as the *letting go* of thoughts and feelings. As my students sit quiet on their mats at the end or beginning of class, I ask them to allow the thoughts and feelings to pass through one after the other. Acknowledge what zips in and out of your brain, but do not pay attention to it. Do not assign it an adjective or tell a story about it. Multiple thoughts can turn to one stream of thought. After a dozen or so breaths, a busy mind will quiet.

Yoga has given us several other, more tangible, ways to guide ourselves into a state of concentration. Here are a few techniques to quiet your mind as you sit in stillness:

Pranayama: Focus on your breath. You can count to yourself. Inhale for 1-2-3 ... Exhale for 3-2-1 ... This will establish a rhythmic breathing pattern; as you continue to sit with only the idea of breath, a buzzing brain will start to settle.

Japa: Repeat a mantra (a sound, chant, or incantation) out loud or in your head. Choose one that fits with your intention — in Sanskrit or otherwise. Or create one of your own. For months my mantra was as simple as book ... love ... yoga ... book ... love ... yoga ... book ... yoga ... love ...

Trataka: Place a lighted candle in front of you. Focus on the flame and try not to blink. Let your vision go blurry and your eyes tear up. Then close your eyes and allow the image of the flame to appear. When you lose the internal image of the flame, open your eyes and concentrate on the flame again. You can go back and forth until you can hold an image of the flame with your eyes closed.

THE COOL DOWN SERIES

"EACH MORNING WE ARE BORN AGAIN.

WHAT WE DO TODAY MATTERS MOST."

—Buddha

14 SUPTA KAPOTASANA
SUPINE PIGEON POSE

Move your body into the pose from *Balasana*:

1 Slowly make your way up to sit on your heels. Slide your hips over to one side and extend your legs out in front. Lie down flat on your back — this is called supine.

2 Bend your knees. Place the soles of your feet on the mat with your heels right in front of your sit bones so that your feet are parallel.

3 Place your right ankle on top of your left knee — the legs look like a #4. Take a breath here.

4 Using the strength of your abdominals, lift the legs up to your chest, keeping the #4 shape. Reach your hands around your left thigh and interlace your fingers. This pose is also called Thread the Needle. Now you can see why.

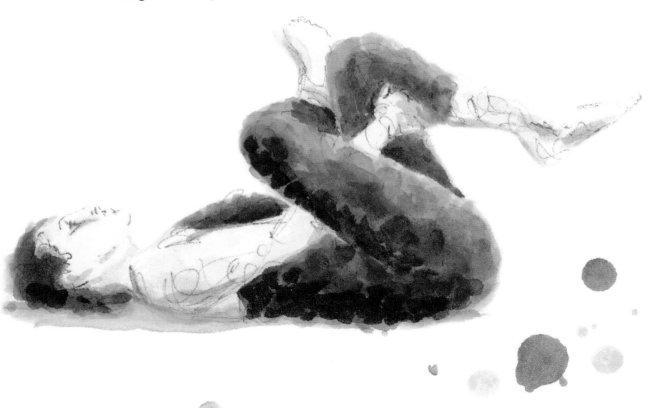

HOW TO PRACTICE

Take FIVE to SEVEN breaths.

If your shoulders have lifted away from the mat, drop them down so the back of your head rests on the mat. As you press the back of your skull into the mat, press your tailbone down to the mat. Feel your back flat.

EXTRA: As your hands draw your left knee closer to your nose, press the right ankle into your knee to bring the right knee away from you. These opposing actions open the hips. Inhale. Draw the left knee in. Exhale. Press the right knee away.

PROP: Grab a strap if your hands don't reach around your thigh. Use one hand on either side of the strap to draw your left knee closer to your nose.

TWO SIDES: Hug your knees into your chest. Rock and roll to massage the muscles of your spine. Then set up for the other side — left ankle over right knee.

THE BENEFITS

MOVE
- stretches the thighs, glutes, psoas, and piriformis muscles
- increases hip flexibility
- relieves back pain

FEEL
- improves self-confidence
- increases creativity
- releases feelings of guilt, worry, and resentments of the past

THINK
- develops reasoning
- calms the brain
- improves executive function

15 SETU BANDHASANA
BRIDGE POSE

Move your body into the pose from *Supta Kapotasana:*

1 Lie down flat on your back —supine.

2 Bend your knees. Place the soles of your feet on the mat with the heels right in front of your sit bones, so that your feet are parallel (just like *Supta Kapotasana*)

3 Reach your arms long by your sides, grab the sides of your mat, with four fingers underneath and thumbs on top. Begin to pull the mat to your toes like you could pull it out from under you. This will open up your chest and shoulders.

4 Press the back of your head into the floor. Press your feet into the floor. Lift your hips.

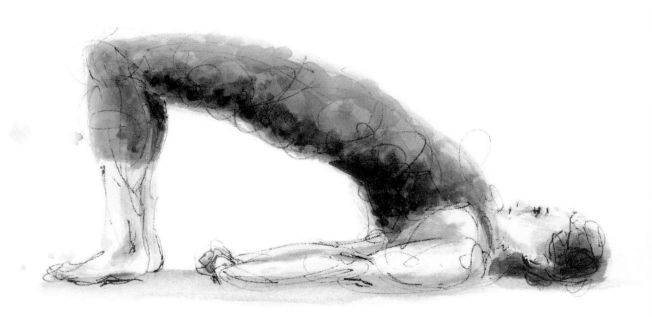

HOW TO PRACTICE

Take FIVE to SEVEN breaths.

Continue to ground down through your arms and feet. Think of reaching your thighs to the front of the mat and reaching your chest to the back of the mat. This will help lengthen your spine.

EXTRA: Keep lifting your hips and pressing your feet down, but let go of the sides of your mat. Start to walk your shoulders together underneath your body. When your hands reach one another, interlace your fingers and bring your palms together. Feel your shoulders open and your chest get broad. Breathe into the space at the front and back of your heart.

PROP: Place a block on the lowest, middle, or highest height (it depends on the flexibility of your spine) underneath your sacrum (the flat part of the lower back above your tailbone). Let the block do the lifting work for you. This is called restorative Bridge Pose. Close your eyes. Stay and breathe as long as you like.

THE BENEFITS

MOVE
- stimulates abdominal organs, lungs, and thyroid
- improves digestion
- reduces back pain, headache, and insomnia

FEEL
- alleviates stress, anxiety, and mild depression
- creates self-awareness
- increases empathy and sympathy

THINK
- calms the central nervous system
- improves communication
- reduces judgment

16 SALAMBA SARVANGASANA
SUPPORTED SHOULDER STAND

Move your body into the pose from
Setu Bandhasana:

1 Lift your hips up and place a block on the lowest or middle height underneath your sacrum. It should feel secure.

2 Bend your knees and lift your feet up. Bring your knees up so that they are right above your hips.

3 Stretch your arms long at your sides — palms facing up.

4 Think about extending through the heel of your foot as you reach one leg up to the ceiling and then the other. Now your heels should be above your hips. It's okay if your legs are not perfectly straight. If you have tight hamstrings, then slightly bend your knees.

HOW TO PRACTICE

Take TEN breaths.

Look straight up at the ceiling — or find a soft gaze between your big toes — to keep your head straight and your neck long. Flex your feet like you are stepping flat on the ceiling. Try to relax the upper half of your body. It's okay if your legs shake. When finished, lower down slowly and lie flat on your back to prevent feeling dizzy after an inversion. These poses reverse the blood flow.

EXTRA: Inhale. Point the right toes to the ceiling. Exhale. Extend the right leg forward as you lower it to hover a few inches above your mat — yes, you will use your abs for this. Inhale. Bring the leg back up to meet with the left. Exhale. Flex the foot. Repeat on the other side. Stop or do less if you feel this in your lower back.

PROP: You're already using a block, but you can make a loop with your strap and fit it around your upper thighs. Pull the strap snug. This will release some of the work your legs have to do to lift up—especially if your legs shake or your hamstrings are tight.

THE BENEFITS

MOVE
- strengthens heart and respiratory system
- decreases varicose veins, reduces wrinkles, and improves complexion
- boosts immune system

FEEL
- energizes
- alleviates anger and frustration
- increases self-expression

THINK
- improves concentration
- decreases fixation
- strengthens intuition

17 PASCHIMOTTANASANA
SEATED FORWARD FOLD

How to move your body into the pose from *Salamba Sarvangasana:*

1 Bring your feet back down to the mat, remove the block, and roll up to sit. Stretch your legs out long in front of you.

2 Press your heels down and bring your big toes to touch. Sit tall to lengthen your spine. Lift your arms straight overhead.

3 Draw your belly back to your spine, which engages the abdominal muscles and protects the lower back. Lift your chest and hinge forward at your hips. Think: Flat back.

4 Walk your hands down either side of your legs and allow your head to drop down. If you can reach your feet, grab your big toes or wrap your fingers around the sides of your feet. If not, place the hands anywhere along the legs. This pose is not about touching your toes.

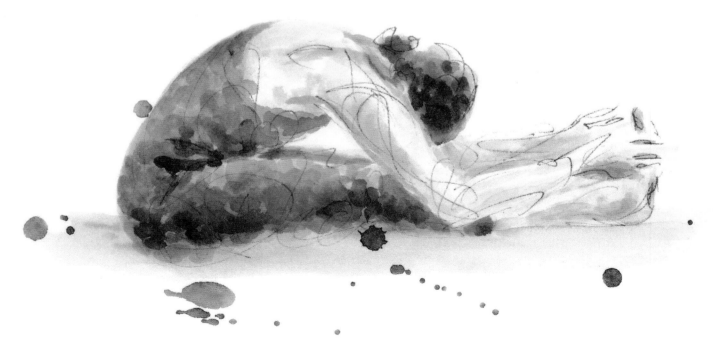

HOW TO PRACTICE

Take FIVE breaths.

If your hamstrings are tight, bend your knees. Make sure to let your head and neck relax to feel the opening from the base of your brain to the base of your tailbone. In Sanskrit this pose means "Intense Stretch of the West" and is designed to open up and lengthen the entire back body. Remember this pose is not about touching your toes.

EXTRA: Bend your knees a lot to relieve tension in the lower back and hamstrings Hug your arms around your shins (or knees) and let your forehead rest on top of your knees. Close your eyes and breathe into your hips and the space at the back of your heart.

PROP: For tight hamstrings, grab a strap. Make sure there are no loops in the strap and place the middle of it around the balls of your feet. Take one side in each hand and begin to fold forward, hinging at your hips.

THE BENEFITS

MOVE
- stretches the muscles along the spine, shoulders, and hamstrings
- regulates appetite
- stimulates liver and kidneys

FEEL
- creates emotional balance
- increases motivation
- strengthens will power

THINK
- reduces mental fatigue
- increases understanding
- improves attention span

18 JANU SIRSASANA
HEAD TO KNEE FORWARD FOLD

How to move your body into the pose from *Paschimottanasana:*

1 Roll one vertebra at a time up to sit tall. Then hug your right knee into your chest, so your right heel gets closer to your right sit bone.

2 Fold your knee out to the right side and press the sole of your right foot into your inner left thigh.

3 Extend your arms up over your head, like *Urdhva Hastasana*. Take a slight twist to the left, to bring your chest over your left knee.

4 Draw your belly back to your spine. Hinge forward at your hips and reach the arms forward, folding down over the left leg. Walk the hands down to the shin or ankle, or around either side of your left foot.

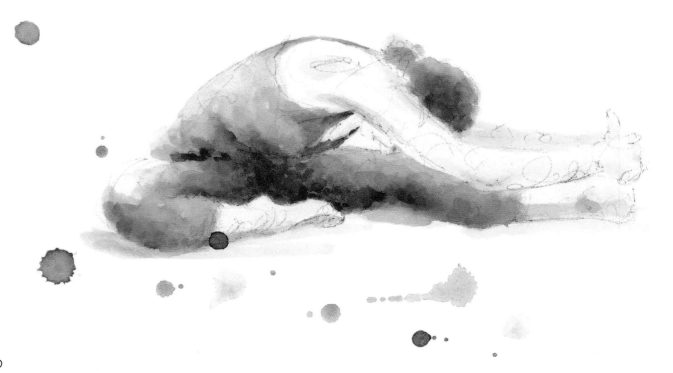

HOW TO PRACTICE

Take FIVE breaths.

Align your belly button over the left knee. Press the heel of your left foot into the floor and reach your toes up, flexing your foot. Let your belly touch first, then your ribs, then your chest, and maybe your nose as you continue to fold forward with a flat, long spine. It's similar to *Paschimottanasana* over your straight leg.

EXTRA: Sit up on a folded blanket to relieve any tension or tightness in the lower back and hamstrings.

PROP: Use a strap around the ball of your left foot. Make sure there is no loop, so you can take either side of the strap in two hands and begin to guide yourself forward over your left leg.

TWO SIDES: Roll up to sit tall. Repeat for FIVE breaths on the other side.

THE BENEFITS

MOVE
- lengthens the waist and the muscles of the lower back
- relieves hypertension, sinusitis, and insomnia
- improves digestion

FEEL
- relieves depression and anxiety
- fosters acceptance
- releases fears

THINK
- improves processing
- calms the brain
- decreases judgment

19 SUPTA MATSYENDRASANA
SUPINE SPINAL TWIST

How to move your body into the pose from *Janu Sirsasana*:

1 Lie down flat on your back. Hug your knees into your chest. Shift your hips an inch or two over to the left and allow your knees to move to the right.

2 As your legs drop down to the floor, try to keep your knees together. Your legs might not reach the floor and that's okay.

3 Reach your arms out to your sides — like a T. Turn your palms up. Relax your legs, your belly, and all the muscles of your back.

4 If it's comfortable for your neck, turn you head to the left. Close your eyes.

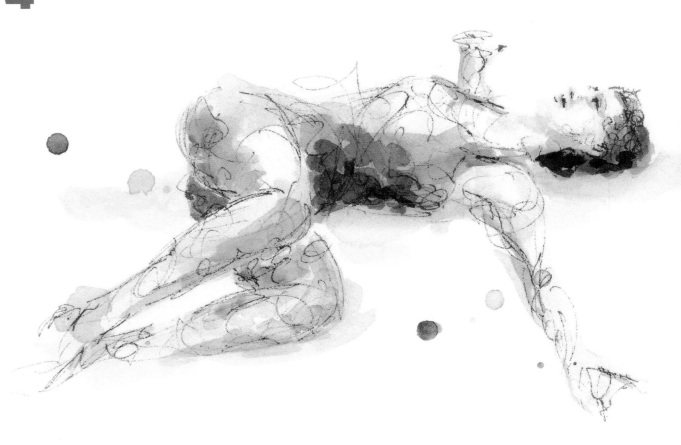

HOW TO PRACTICE

Take FIVE to TEN breaths.

Don't worry too much if your shoulders or knees don't reach to the mat or floor. Close your eyes. Breathe deep into the belly. Release through the entire body and let gravity do the work.

EXTRA: Slide the right leg out from under the left. Place the right ankle on top of the left knee. Let the legs sink back down to the floor, letting gravity do the work.

PROP: If your legs do not rest together comfortably, take a folded blanket (or a block) and place it between your knees. Then release into the twist.

TWO SIDES: Hug both knees back into center. Repeat on the left side and hold for FIVE to TEN breaths.

THE BENEFITS

MOVE
- tones the waistline
- lubricates the spinal discs and realigns the spine
- massages internal organs and removes toxins

FEEL
- alleviates emotional stress
- energizes
- reduces anger

THINK
- improves problem solving
- clears the mind
- creates self-awareness

20 SAVASANA
CORPSE POSE

How to move your body into the pose from *Supta Matsyendrasana*:

1 Stretch your legs out straight. Let your toes flop out. Feel your heels, legs, and hips sinking down into the earth.

2 Stretch your arms long at your sides. Let your palms face up. Feel your arms, shoulders, and the back of your head sinking down into the earth.

3 Close your eyes.

4 Breathe.

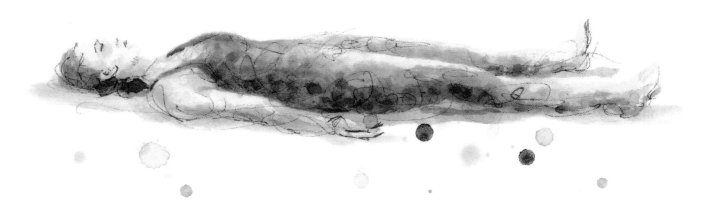

HOW TO PRACTICE

Stay in Savasana for FOUR to SEVEN MINUTES.

As you lie still, concentrate on your breath. Deepen your exhales. Deepen your inhales. Resist the urge to move or resituate. Sometimes the most challenging thing to do is be still. Allow your mind to be calm. You don't need to block any thoughts but don't let them stick. Acknowledge what is passing through your brain, but let it go. This pose is about total release and rejuvenation. Don't worry if you fall asleep — it's cool, it happens to all of us.

EXTRA: Inhale. Send the breath to the base of your spine. Exhale. ... Inhale. Send the breath to your hips. Exhale. ... Inhale. Send the breath to your belly. Exhale. ... Inhale. Send the breath to your heart. Exhale. ... Inhale. Send the breath to your throat. Exhale. ... Inhale. Send the breath to the space between your eyebrows. Exhale. ... Inhale. Send the breath to the crown of your head. Exhale.

PROP: If your lower back is tight or you have lower back pain, place a rolled up blanket underneath your knees.

THE BENEFITS

THE BENEFITS OF THIS POSE ARE ENDLESS. MAKE SURE YOU TAKE THE TIME TO STAY FOR AT LEAST THREE MINUTES. BUT KNOW THAT SEVEN WILL MAKE A BIGGER DIFFERENCE. SOME DAYS *SAVASANA* IS EASY. SOME DAYS IT IS MORE CHALLENGING. BUT AS MUCH AS YOU ARE TEMPTED TO, DO NOT SKIP THIS POSE. I WILL SAY IT AGAIN – THE BENEFITS OF *SAVASANA* ARE ENDLESS.

DHYANA

PRACTICE MEDITATION:

DYANA IS THE STATE OF UNINTERRUPTED CONCENTRATION.

It goes one step further than *dharana*. The mind is aware without having to focus.

The practice of *dhyana* does not come overnight. Many things — those last six limbs of yoga — have to fall into place before the body is able to sit in stillness and the mind is able to clear. The outer and inner worlds have been calmed by the *yamas* and the *niyamas*. The body is ready for stillness from the practice of *asana* and *pranayama*. The senses have been quieted with the practice of *pratyahara*. The mind is clear from practicing *dharana*. Only now is one ready for next stage of meditation or *dhyana*.

Dhyana is the limb of yoga in which the mind is without thoughts. Empty. Completely devoid of opinions, contemplations, and emotions. There is no place for words or reasoning or explanation. There is no longer a sense of self to connect to. This limb is quite tricky, and even the wisest of sages acknowledges how challenging it can be to reach *dhyana* — an exalted state of oneness.

Yoga teachers call this idea of dropping into meditation "finding your seat." And it is entirely possible to find your seat and then lose it again over and over and over. But when you find it, you will know. Whether you are sitting on a fancy meditation pillow beside a window or on a park bench or cross-legged on your mat in yoga class with dozens of others, you will know. People describe it in a myriad of ways. Like they are floating above the ground. Seeing patterns of light. Swaying. Experiencing overwhelming emotions. Tingles.

Here is a bit of what happens in your brain. The frontal lobe (reasoning, executive functioning, decision making) goes quiet. The parietal lobe (processing sensory information, orienting in time and space) slows way down. The thalamus (sensory perception, bringing the outside world in) greatly reduces the influx of information. Reticular formation (flight or flight, arousal, reaction) dials down.

The idea is that we take a moment — a few minutes, or a few hours — to tap out of our lives. We go somewhere else and that somewhere is different for everyone. But it is somewhere that is calm and allows for peace and enlightenment. After some practice, you will notice the signs that signal that you're on your way to your seat, to the meditative state of *dhyana*. In my personal practice, my body starts to sway with my breath. I feel a subtle tingling sensation. Sometimes my inner world washes over in purple. And I'm on my way to the place where time elapses, where my brain clears, and where my heart opens.

There is no right or wrong way to experience meditation. All you need is a quiet place and an intention to concentrate — on breath or mantra or light or sound. Sit and see where it takes you.

THE EIGHTH LIMB OF YOGA

SAMADHI

PRACTICE ENLIGHTENMENT: SAMADHI IS ANOTHER REALM.

It is the esoteric world that lies beyond our waking, sleeping, dreaming world.

Samadhi is the pinnacle of meditation. The body and senses are at rest, but the mind remains sharp and alert. When you are experiencing *Samadhi*, with the physical body acting as if it has gone to sleep (at rest) and the mental body supremely alert (*dhyana*), you are in a state that is beyond consciousness.

There is no longer an attachment to the physical world around you. There is no longer an attachment to the self. There is only a universal consciousness. There is truth. There is joy. Some yogis call this stage *ananda,* which means bliss.

In *Light on Yoga,* B.K.S Iyengar describes this final stage on the yogic path.

> "There is a peace that passeth all understanding. The mind cannot find words to describe the state and the tongue fails to utter them. The state can only be expressed by profound silence. The yogi has departed from the material world and merged in the eternal."

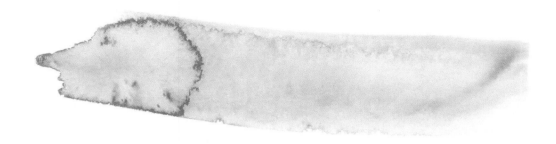

Chances are that whole concept of "going beyond" is hard to grasp. I had a student who gave me a taste of what this might be like for another person. He had just begun his yoga practice. He was both flexible and strong. As we moved through the *asanas* together, he grew frustrated, asked questions, proved his physical strength, and more than he needed to, tested his will power. In short, he was ambitious. Yet in *Savasana*, he was like no other student I've ever taught. *He got it.* He let go of every muscle, every thought, every everything. He was the epitome of what I say when I say "just let everything you hear, see, feel, and experience melt into one puddle of existence." This is the essence of final rest.

"That's [*Savasana*] my favorite one," he'd say when we were finished with the sessions. One day I asked him why, and he told me that he just lets his body go and that (on this particular day) he started thinking about a river in Wyoming he once visited. "It was the only thought in my mind, that river," he said. *One-pointed concentration,* I thought. "And then nothing else in my mind seems to matter. I just go to this other place. I don't even think about that river. I just don't think. But I'm not asleep either. I mean I know I'm not asleep, but I'm not awake."

And the truth of it is, it doesn't matter where he goes. And to be honest, not everyone can just drop into relaxation quite the way this man can. Yet, just like it doesn't matter if you can or can't do that crazy arm balance or stand on your head for five minutes or touch your toes, it doesn't matter if we fall in and out of the states of concentration, meditation, and bliss.

THE EIGHT-LIMBED PATH OF YOGA WILL TAKE YOU EXACTLY WHERE YOU NEED TO GO. AND WHERE YOU GO WILL MATTER TO NO ONE ELSE BUT YOU.

MOVE · FEEL · THINK
SEQUENCE

Now that you have made it through every pose, here is the entire MOVE FEEL THINK sequence. Now you can practice this *Vinyasa* flow—Warm up to Cool Down—one pose after the other. As you move through each *asana*, I invite you to keep in mind a few things:

BREATH: Find an even breath throughout. You can count for 5 breaths or 2 or 9. As you breathe, inhale and exhale out through your nose. Practice *Ujjayi* breath.

PACE: Go at your own speed. Each day can be different. There might even be some poses you want to stay in longer than others. This is your practice, so there is no one there to rush you or make you stay too long.

SPACE: Learn to hold your own space when you practice. Make enough room for you and your mat. Put on music or light a candle if that feels right. **Turn off your phone.**

AWARENESS: If we all did every yoga pose right, there would be nothing to practice and to learn from. Seek compassoin in each pose, knowing that some will come easier than others. Listen to the feedback from your brain and body. Experience sensation, but do not put yourself in pain.

PRESENCE: You be you. That's a line I took from a great teacher and friend. You be you. This practice is about getting to know who you are today, in the moment, on your mat. That may ebb and flow and change, but it will never be anyone but who you are today.

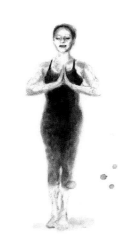

5 BREATHS

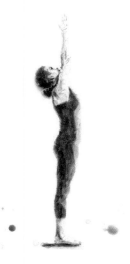

INHALE

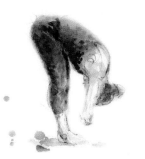

EXHALE

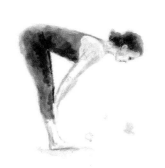

INHALE

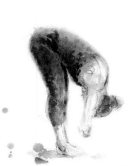

EXHALE

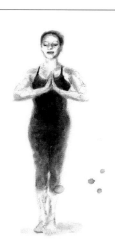

INHALE

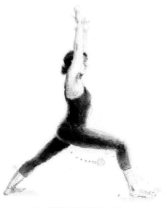

3 BREATHS
BOTH SIDES

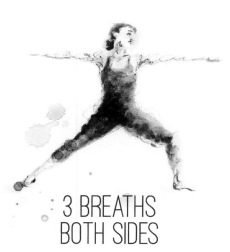

3 BREATHS
BOTH SIDES

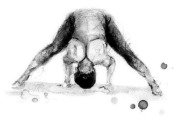

5 BREATHS

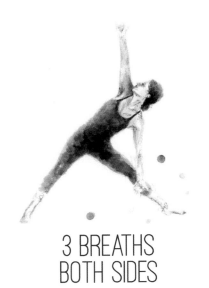

3 BREATHS
BOTH SIDES

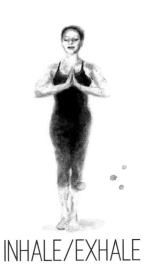

INHALE/EXHALE

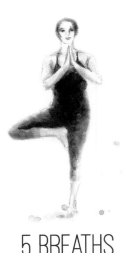

5 BREATHS
BOTH SIDES

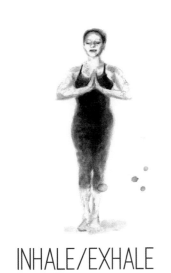

INHALE/EXHALE

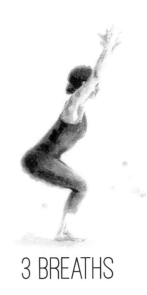

3 BREATHS

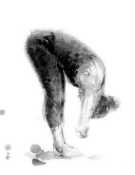

EXHALE

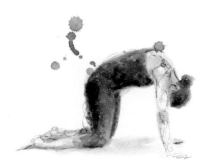

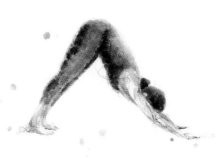

CAT/COW UNDULATIONS

5 BREATHS

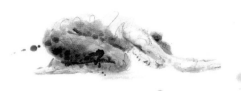 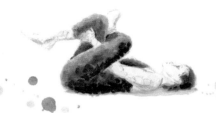 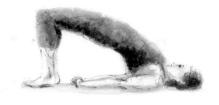

5 BREATHS   5 BREATHS   3 BREATHS
                   BOTH SIDES

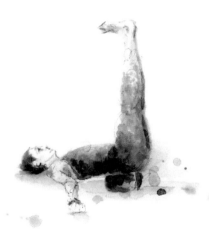 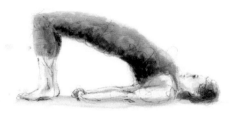 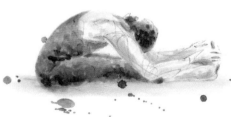

7 BREATHS   3 BREATHS   5 BREATHS

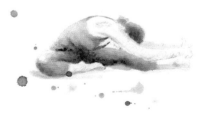 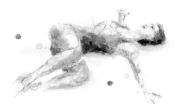 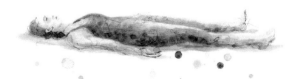

5 BREATHS   5 BREATHS   5 MINUTES
BOTH SIDES   BOTH SIDES

THE SEVEN CHAKRAS

I know
SAHASRARA
space
Chant silent *OM* CROWN CHAKRA

universal consciousness
transcendence
being

7

I see
ANJA
THIRD EYE CHAKRA **light**
Chant *OM*

clarity
imagination
visualization

6

5

I speak
VISHUDDHA
sound
Chant *HAM* THROAT CHAKRA

truth
communication
independence

4

love
passion
devotion

I love
ANAHATA
air
Chant *YAM* HEART CHAKRA

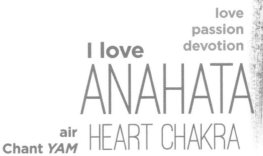

stability
survival
purification

MULADHARA **I am**

ROOT CHAKRA **earth**
Chant *LAM*

1

2

I feel SVADISTHANA

creativity SACRAL CHAKRA **water**
sensuality **Chant *VAM***
intimacy

3

power
transformation
self-esteem

MANIPURA **I do**
SOLAR PLEXUS CHAKRA

fire
Chant *RAM*

GLOSSARY/TERMS

abduction: the movement of a limb away from the midline of the body

adduction: the movement of a limb toward the midline of the body

ananda: the condition of utter joy; bliss

asana: physical posture; the third limb of yoga

behavioral: of or relating to an individual's reactions, emotions, and behaviors

brahmari: bee breath

chakra: a psycho-energetic center of the subtle body

cognitive: of or relating to an individual's mental activity, thought processing and understanding

coronal plane: divides the body from front to back; movement along this plane are adduction and abduction

dharana: concentration; the sixth limb of yoga

dhyana: meditation; the seventh limb of yoga

drishti: a soft gaze

executive function: set of mental processes that helps connect past experience with present action; activities such as planning, organizing, strategizing, paying attention to and remembering details, and managing time and space.

extension: a movement that increases the angle between two body parts

flexion: a movement that decreases the angle between two body parts

japa: the spoken repetition of mantra

kapalbhati: breath of fire

mantra: chant; incantation

mudra: hand gesture; seal

nadi shodhana: alternative nostril breath

namaste: the light in me salutes and honors the light within you

niyama: inward observances; the second limb of yoga

om (aum): the sound of the universe

padmasana: lotus pose

parivrtta: revolved; twisted

PTSD: can occur after someone goes through a traumatic event like combat, assault, or disaster

prana: breath; life force

pranayama: rhythmic control of breath; the fourth limb of yoga

pratyahara: withdrawal of the senses; detachment; the fifth limb of yoga

proprioception: awareness of the body in space

sagittal plane: divides the body from right to left; movements along this plane are abduction and adduction

samadhi: enlightenment; bliss; the eighth limb of yoga

sat: truth; ultimate reality

simhasana: lion's breath

sthira: strength; steadiness

subtle body: the energetic body

sukha: joy; ease

sukhasana: easy pose

supine: flat on one's back

supta: reclined; supine; sleeping

surya namaskar: sun salutation

tapas: heat; energy; to burn

transverse plane: divides the body from top to bottom; movements along this plane are rotations

trataka: candle gazing

trauma: a deeply distressing or disturbing experience; an incident or injury that causes an individual to experience physical or emotional symptoms

ujjayi: victorious breath; oceanic breath

utthita: extended

vinyasa: to put or place in a special way; synchronizes breath to movement

yama: outward observances; the first limb of yoga

yoga sutra: aphorism; thread

FURTHER READING AND RESOURCES

Here are a dozen books, from the most obviously yogic to a more the off the mat way to see the practice.

The Yoga Sutras of Pantanjali translation by Swami Satchidinanda
The Bhagavad Gita translation by Eknath Easwaran
Light on Yoga B.K.S. Iyengar
The Heart of Yoga T.K.V. Desikachar
The Key Muscles of Yoga Ray Long
Yoga as Medicine Timothy McCall
Buddha's Brain Rick Hanson
Fierce Medicine Ana T. Forrest
The Brain That Changes Itself Norman Doidge
When Things Fall Apart Pema Chodron
The Four Agreements Miguel Ruiz
He Never Liked Cake Janna Leyde

Yoga themed websites are plentiful, but these six will get you started on your quest for more inspiration, interesting articles, information, anecdotes, and many more yoga book suggestions.

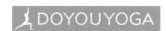

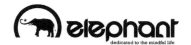

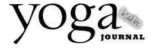

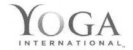

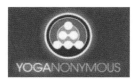

ACKNOWLEDGEMENTS

Dear reader, thank you for picking up this book. You may have endured trauma, you may teach yoga, or you may know nothing of either, but I am grateful to share this practice with you.

I want to acknowledge those who have supported Move Feel Think on pubslush.com, those of you are on the Namaste List.

I also want to acknowledge and thank those of who have influenced my yoga practice and supported my teaching. Kevin, Kim and Ashleigh, who were yoga teachers at Hearst in 2009. Nessi Erkmenoglu, for buying me a Jivamukti class pass for my birthday. My beautifully knowledgeable and inspiring teachers at Sonic Yoga—Johanna Bell, Tracy Mohr, Lauren Hanna, Jeffrey Duval, and Dan Wilf. My Sonic Yoga Teacher Training class of Spring 2011, for our many weeks and hours on (and off) the mat together. The Mala Yoga Community, for strengthening my teaching and setting my foundation, for encouraging me to go forth and find my voice, be confident in what I know, develop this practice, and write this book. Jennifer Whitney, Daniella Rosales-Friedman, and Anna Greenberg, for all you have taught me as teachers and friends. Lindsay Sullivan, for classes, coffees, and for introducing me to the power of Jupiter and Thursdays. Emily Leonardo, for rolling out a mat next to me more times than we can count. Christina Hatgis, for teaching me how to engage in Down Dog, for all the times I subbed your basics classes. Angela Clark, for suggesting that blogs could become a book, for our few practice sequences. Steph Creaturo, for coffees, for your classes, for your words, for your support, and for helping me navigate who I am as a teacher. Hilary Hudgins and Shenaaz Jetha, for the wild support you give me and this endeavor. Oscar Aguilera, for making teaching to Wounded Warriors possible. Erika Beras for NPR. "Dr. Joe" Pecorelli, thank you for encouraging my father to practice and for me to participate. Maryellen Romero, for our belief and your words. BIAPA, for the audience and the microphone. The team at ReMed, for trusting and believing in this. I also want to thank and acknowledge my friends and family for your love support and listening ears for "book #2." Abby Ludwig, for your compassion in the early years and for our pilot program and our friendship. Anna Gilbert Zupon, for our chats that remind me why we do this and how to stay to true to who we are. Mary Holahan Myles and Kate Geller, for listening to me talk this out over and over, for practicing with me, for being my wild support in Pittsburgh. Sarah Reiber and Krystal Renszel, for believing in this—both personally and professionally. Lauren Berger, for being my teacher-training pincushion and the editor who killed my darlings. Chad Hockenjos, for your love and patience on one too many stressful days, for understanding what this means to me, and for practicing these poses, irfly. Emily Balawejder, you have created magic with my words and Nicole's art, so I cannot thank you enough for your design and for making this book into something even more beautiful than I could have ever imagined. Nicole Ryan, for your time and patience, for sharing your incredible talent with me to illustrate this book, and for also killing some darlings, DKF. Mom, for giving me the idea, for Morning Cup of Yoga, for the many printouts you gave Dad to help him practice, for reading and talking about a lot of stuff you were unfamiliar with, and for your unwavering encouragement. Dad, for 'driveway yoga,' for helping me see this practice of yoga in a whole new light, for teaching me when I thought I was teaching you, and for practicing with me. My students, you have no idea how much I learn from you, how much I love sharing this practice with you. Thank you for showing up. Yoga, for existing and for transcending time and space and what I struggle to understand.

NAMASTE LIST

Maryellen Romero, Jessica Shenker, Lauren Berger, Ken DuVilla, Claudia Leyde, John Leyde, Dina Stubert Landfried, Danielle Henderson, Annie Carlin, Margaret Leyde, Jean Leyde, Julie Weber, Justine Schofield, George Jones, Didi Gluck, Barb Connelly, Larry Connelly, Annie Abraham, Alejandra Serret, Patti Schmitt, Nicole Breyette, Lauren Feighan, Danny Rieg, William Hunnell, Maggie Ornstein, Andrea Berger, Michael Berger, Jennifer Makowski, Lynn Ellenberger, Joanne Jackal, Kate Durie, Katie Karlson, Richard Gartner, Jeannie Lengenfelder Brenner, Claire Harmon, Sarah Reiber, Donna Creed, Jodie Mount, Samantha Watson, Kate Levin, Helen Phillips, Amelie Walker, Emily Balawejder, Krystal Renszel, Anusha Alikhan, Kate Geller, Barb Dively, Mary Holahan, Duke Chandler, Leta Koontz, Dustin Buss, Mala Yoga, Lori Williams, Jessica Gernhardt, Elizabeth McCaffrey, Sara Mendelson, Anna Guest-Jelley, Hilary Hudgins, Emily Cantin, Carolyn Gallo, Paula Thomas, Theresa Bond, Jake Yale, Sarah DeRoy, Rosemary Rawlins, Michelle Versaw, Vicky Suhrie, Michael Madonia, Natalie King

Printed in Great Britain
by Amazon